Juta's Introduction to Paediatric Surgical Nursing

Editors
Sophie Mogotlane & Mokgadi Matlakala

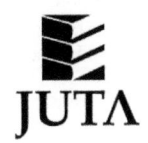

JUTA

Disclaimer

In the writing of this book, every effort has been made to present accurate and up-to-date information from the best and most reliable sources. However, the results of healthcare professionals depend on a variety of factors that are beyond the control of the authors and publishers. Therefore, neither the authors nor the publishers assume responsibility for, nor make any warranty with regard to, the outcomes achieved from the procedures described in this book.

The authors and publisher have exerted every effort to ensure that drug selections and dosages set forth in this text are in accord with current recommendations and practice at the time of publication. However, readers are urged to check the package insert for each drug for any change in indications of dosage and for added warning and precautions. The information in this book is provided in good faith and the authors and publisher cannot be held responsible for errors, individual responses to drugs and other consequences.

Juta's Introduction to Paediatric Surgical Nursing

First published 2018

Juta and Company (Pty) Ltd
First floor, Sunclare building, 21 Dreyer street, Claremont 7708
PO Box 14373, Lansdowne 7779, Cape Town, South Africa
www.juta.co.za

© 2018 Juta and Company (Pty) Ltd

ISBN 978 1 48511 576 2

All rights reserved. No part of this publication may be reproduced or transmitted in any form or by any means, electronic or mechanical, including photocopying, recording, or any information storage or retrieval system, without prior permission in writing from the publisher. Subject to any applicable licensing terms and conditions in the case of electronically supplied publications, a person may engage in fair dealing with a copy of this publication for his or her personal or private use, or his or her research or private study. See section 12(1)(a) of the Copyright Act 98 of 1978.

Project manager: Carlyn Bartlett-Cronje
Editor: Sarah Koopman
Proofreader: Christa Büttner-Rohwer
Cover designer: Genevieve Simpson
Typesetter: Wouter Reinders
Indexer: Derika van Biljon

Typeset in 9.5 pt on 12 pt Optima Lt Std

The author and the publisher believe on the strength of due diligence exercised that this work does not contain any material that is the subject of copyright held by another person. In the alternative, they believe that any protected pre-existing material that may be comprised in it has been used with appropriate authority or has been used in circumstances that make such use permissible under the law.

Contents

Preface	**iii**
Section 1: Introduction to child care	**1**
Chapter 1: Introduction to child care	**3**
Introduction	6
Growth and development	6
Factors that influence growth and development in child care	*7*
Normal milestones in a child's development	*8*
Conclusion	11
References	12
Chapter 2: Reactions of a child to hospitalisation	**13**
Introduction	14
Reaction of a child to hospitalisation	15
Reaction of parents to the child's hospitalisation	16
Reaction of siblings to hospitalisation	16
Management of siblings	*17*
Assessment and common findings	17
Subjective data	*17*
Objective data	*18*
Assisting the child to adapt in hospital	18
The role of parents	*18*
Sibling participation	*18*
Child's participation in own care	*19*
Pain in children	19
Principles of pain assessment in children	*19*
Questioning the child about pain	*20*
Questioning parents about the child's pain	*20*
Pain rating scales	*20*
Responses when in pain	*21*
Conclusion	21
References	21
Section 2: Introduction to surgical nursing in child care	**23**
Chapter 3: Nursing care of a child in the pre-operative period	**25**
Introduction	27
Indications for surgery	28
Suffixes used to describe surgical procedures	28

Classification and types of surgery	28
The needs of a child who is to undergo surgery	29
Nursing assessment and common findings in a patient to undergo surgery	30
Subjective data	*31*
Objective data	*32*
Preoperative care	32
Preoperative risk factors	*33*
Legal and ethical issues in preoperative care	34
Informed consent for operation	*34*
Legal requirements for a valid consent	*35*
The day of surgery	37
Transportation of the patient from the ward to the operating theatre	*37*
Conclusion	38
References	39
Chapter 4: Intraoperative nursing care of children	**41**
Introduction	42
The theatre environment	42
The intraoperative care team	43
The role of the theatre reception nurse	44
The role of the scrub nurse	45
The role of the circulating nurse	45
The role of the anaesthetic nurse	46
Reception of the patient in the operating room	46
Positioning the patient on the operating table	47
Induction of anaesthesia	47
Recovery room care	48
Return to the ward and handover	49
Intraoperative complications	49
During the operation	*49*
In the recovery room	*50*
Conclusion	53
References	54
Chapter 5: Postoperative nursing care of children	**55**
Introduction	56
Preparation of the environment	57
Immediate care on arrival in the ward	57
Common postoperative problems	*58*
Subsequent care	59
Late postoperative-period nursing care	61
Late postoperative complications	*61*
Complications of wound healing	*61*
Preparation for discharge and essential health information	62
Conclusion	67
References	67

Section 3: Common surgical conditions in children **69**
Chapter 6: Surgical conditions of the face: cleft lip and cleft palate **71**
   Introduction 72
   Congenital defects of the face 72
      Cleft lip 72
      Subjective data 73
      Objective data 73
      Cleft palate 75
   Conclusion 80
   References 80
Chapter 7: Congenital defects of the gastrointestinal tract system **81**
   Introduction 82
   Congenital defects of the oesophagus and the trachea 83
      Oesophageal atresia and tracheo-oesophageal fistula 83
      Types of oesophageal and tracheo-oesophageal defects 83
      Clinical manifestations of oesophageal defects 83
      Preoperative care of a child with oesophageal atresia with or without tracheal fistula 84
      Postoperative care of a child who has undergone repair of oesophageal defects with or without a tracheal fistula 87
   Congenital diaphragmatic hernia 91
      Management of congenital diaphragmatic hernia 92
      Postoperative care 92
   Hypertrophic pyloric stenosis 96
      Clinical manifestations 96
      Management 97
      Specific preoperative care 97
      Specific postoperative care 97
   Intussusception 98
      Types of intussusception 98
      Clinical manifestations 99
      Assessment findings 99
      Management of intussusception 99
      Specific preoperative care 99
      Specific postoperative care 100
   Volvulus 100
      Specific preoperative care 101
      Specific postoperative care 101
   Congenital aganglionic megacolon (Hirschsprung's disease) 101
      Clinical manifestations 102
      Specific preoperative care 103
      Specific postoperative care 103
   Imperforate anus 103
      Clinical manifestations 103
      Assessment and common findings 103
      Management 104

Specific postoperative care... 104
Hernias... 104
   Types of hernias 104
Conclusion... 110
Reference 111

Section 4: Inflammatory surgical conditions 113
Chapter 8: Acute appendicitis and appendicectomy 115
Introduction 116
   Management of appendicitis.. 117
Potential complications of appendicitis that might impact negatively on the surgery (appendicectomy)... 118
Conclusion... 120
References 120

Chapter 9: Tonsillitis, tonsillectomy and adenoidectomy............................ 121
Introduction 122
Assessment and common findings.. 122
Preoperative care.. 122
Postoperative care following tonsillectomy... 123
Essential patient teaching 124
Peritonsillar abscess (quinsy).. 124
Care of a child with tracheostomy 126
   Indications for a tracheostomy... 126
   Potential problems of a tracheostomy 126
   Principles of tracheostomy care 127
Conclusion... 127
References 128

Chapter 10: The child and trauma: fractures 129
Introduction 130
Clinical manifestations of a fracture... 131
Bone healing in children.. 131
Management of a fracture 132
Reduction of the fracture... 133
   Specific preoperative care.. 133
Postoperative care 136
Complications of a fracture 136
Amputation... 137
   Specific preoperative care.. 137
   Specific postoperative care.. 137
Conclusion... 141
References 142

Chapter 11: Surgical conditions of the central nervous system: hydrocephalus 143
Introduction 144
Types of hydrocephalus 144
Specific preoperative care 146
Specific postoperative care 147

Complications of shunts 147
Discharge plan 147
    Family health education 147
Conclusion 148
References 148

Addendum A: Guidelines on basic care provisions in surgical wards and paediatric units 149
Checklist for PO5 Surgical Ward 151
Checklist for PO6 Paediatric Ward 162

Preface

Over the years, child nursing has become a speciality based on many emergent pathogens and social issues, and the realisation of how these impact on child care. Research conducted on child care has also increased the awareness of family as the main partner in child care and the major role families have to play in child care. This is an introductory text to paediatric surgical nursing to further create that space in caring and provide the necessary attention to common surgical conditions in child care in basic nursing. Paediatric surgical nursing conditions, such as tetralogy of Fallot, spina bifida, hydrocephalus and shunts, and others in the same league, requiring advanced specialist nursing care, are beyond the scope of this text.

An ill child who has to be hospitalised for whatever reason is more concerned about separation than the circumstances that brought her or him to hospital. So, in the care provided, more time has to be set aside to allow for adaptation to the hospital environment. At this stage the family will play a major role in helping the child to settle in as it is best positioned to do this.

The text is limited to paediatric surgical nursing for undergraduate nurses. In recent years, with advances in medicine, surgery is limited to correction of congenital defects that are life-threatening and function limiting, and to repair and/or reduction of acquired defects that will not spontaneously heal or reduce. Many inflammatory conditions that were previously managed by surgical means (including abscesses) are now treated with antibiotics.

The text will therefore provide the nurse with knowledge and basic skill to care for children with common surgical conditions that can be managed in the nursery or general ward and not in the intensive care unit.

In the wake of National Health Insurance (NHI), the text includes two addenda, P05 and P06, which provide guidelines on elements of basic care in a surgical ward or a paediatric unit.

The Editor
Sophie M. Mogotlane

Section 1

Introduction to child care

1 Introduction to child care

LEARNING OBJECTIVES

On completion of this Chapter, you should be able to:
- describe growth and development as it applies to child care
- explain the factors that influence growth and development in child care
- outline the child's milestones in growth and development.

KEY CONCEPTS AND TERMINOLOGY

adaptation:	The body's adjustment to and accommodation of environmental factors to maintain stability.
cephalo-caudal:	A term used to describe a child's development from the head to the toe. In growth and development, the child needs to develop the neck muscles that hold the head steady before the back can be strong to allow the child to sit and progress to stand and walk. It is only when the child can sit and sometimes stand and walk that toilet training can commence.
child:	According to the South African Children's Act 38 of 2005, in line with the United Nations, a child is anyone under the age of 18. The term is inclusive of neonate, infant and adolescent.
childhood morbidity:	This is the incidence of ill health in children from birth to 5 years.
child mortality:	The death of infants and children under the age of 5 years in a given year per 1000 children in this age group.
development:	An increase in complexity of function and progression of skills.
due date:	This is the expected date of the delivery of a full-term baby on or after 38 weeks of gestation.
foetus:	This is a stage of development of a human being after 2 months of fertilisation until birth.
full-term infant:	A baby born between 38 and 42 weeks of gestation.
gametes:	A mature haploid male or female germ cell which is able to unite with another of the opposite sex in sexual reproduction to form a zygote.
growth:	The increase in size as determined by muscle bulk, weight, height, and increase in bone and organ size.

infant:	A general term to refer to a newborn, a young child or baby. The term is used to address a child in the period from birth to 12 months.
infant mortality rate:	This is the number of deaths within a specific population during the first year of life per 1000 live births.
large-for-dates:	This is an infant who is overgrown as determined by weight, which may be above expectation for the gestational age before or at birth. This may be due to maternal diabetes mellitus and/or other congenital defects such as erythroblastosis fetalis and transposition of the great blood vessels.
live birth:	This refers to an infant who shows signs of life after delivery (heartbeat, respiration, movement) regardless of gestation period and weight at birth.
lodger mother:	This refers to a mother who is allowed to stay with the child in hospital and participates in the child's care in the ward.
low birth weight:	These are infants who weigh between 1 kg and 2.5 kg at full-term birth.
maturation:	The term relates to sequential physical changes as a result of growth and development.
milestone:	This is a significant event to mark a change or stage in a child's development. Milestones are a series of sequential events that mark achievements in the child's growth and development.
neonatal mortality rate:	The number of deaths that occur in the first month of birth per 1000 live births in a specific population.
neonatal period:	This is the first 28 days after birth. It is further subdivided into the early neonatal period, which is the first 7 days post delivery, which overlaps with the perinatal period and late neonatal period, which commences on the 8th day post delivery and concludes on the 28th day.
operation:	In this context, the term refers to the performance of a surgical procedure. In general terms, operation is synonymous to surgery.
paediatrics:	The branch of medicine concerned with the development, care, diseases and disease management of infants, children and adolescents.
perinatal mortality rate:	This includes stillbirths and early neonatal deaths and is expressed per 1000 total births in a specific population.

perinatal period:	This is the period from the 22nd week of pregnancy to the end of the first week of life after birth.
pincer grip:	The ability of a child to hold objects between the index finger and the thumb.
poly-hydramnios:	An accumulation of amniotic fluid during pregnancy.
post-term infant:	This is a baby born after the 42nd week of gestation.
preterm/premature infants:	These are infants who are born before the 37th week (259 days) of gestation.
proximo-distal:	A term used to describe the development of a child from the centre outward. For example, a child has to develop strong chest muscles and arms before he can crawl or achieve the pincer grip.
small-for-dates:	This is an infant whose growth was retarded in utero due to intrauterine infections of the mother, or placental insufficiency and may be born before, at or after the due date of birth.
stillbirth:	An infant who, after 22 weeks of gestation, exhibits no signs of life at birth.
stillbirth rate:	This is the number of stillbirths per 1000 births in a specific population. In developed countries the rate is 3 per 1000 births, while in underdeveloped or developing countries the rate is 28 per 1000 births.
surgery:	In this context, the term surgery refers to the performance of an operation. In general terms, surgery is synonymous with operation.
trimester:	This is the three-monthly management of pregnancy. The first three months are referred to as the first trimester, the second grouping of three months as the second trimester, and the last three months as the last trimester.
zygote:	A multicellular organism formed from a fertilisation event between two gametes.

PREREQUISITE KNOWLEDGE

- Human anatomy and physiology, biophysics and biochemistry
- Social sciences
- Family and community health.

MEDICO-LEGAL CONSIDERATIONS

Paediatrics is a specialised study of children, both in health and in disease. Children are often prone to hazards and this must be kept in mind in their care. The child's age, weight and health status must always be taken into consideration when calculating dosages for medication and planning for treatment, as overdosage and/or underdosage can occur inadvertently. The skin may be irritated and disintegrate with the use of the mildest of chemicals because the child's skin is delicate and the immune system is immature.

ETHICAL CONSIDERATIONS

Involvement of parents and/or caregivers is very important in child care. In some instances where the child is old enough it may be necessary to get her or him involved. It is important to provide caregivers with information that will help them understand the activities that take place around the child. The child must also be informed about what is happening to his body and why it is happening. The outcomes of treatment must be explained without overestimation and without raising the parents' hope unduly. The child must be treated with respect and commitment regardless of age.

ESSENTIAL HEALTH LITERACY

Child care is a very rewarding but labour-intensive experience. Parental involvement is always helpful because they are better able to comfort the child when the child is stressed. It is important for health practitioners to provide parents with information that will enable them to participate in the care and make a meaningful contribution. Parents need to understand the link between the milestones and child's behaviour. For example, parents must know that only when the child can stand will they be able to comply to toilet training (cephalo-caudal). Parents need to understand the anatomy, physiology, and the physical, social and emotional development of children and that children are human beings with minds of their own. They must provide the necessary support and protection and allow the child to explore their environment within safety limits. They must instil discipline and must exhibit it with care, confidence and love.

Introduction

The growth and development of a child occurs from conception. It is an ongoing dynamic process throughout life. It is sequential and is influenced by hereditary and environmental factors such as genes, family, parents, peers, society, culture, values, customs, societal rules and resources.

Growth and development

In child care, the terms growth and development are usually used interchangeably and together. It is not possible to refer to one without the other. They both occur in an orderly and sequential manner within the child's milestones, whereupon development of skill allows the child to increasingly respond to the environment.

Growth relates to increase in size as measured in height, weight, head circumference, or any parts of the body, such as bones and organs. The increase can be measured quantitatively. At birth the average height ranges between 48 cm and 54 cm, weight ranges between 2.7 kg and 3.8 kg, head circumference ranges between 33 cm and 37 cm (Harrison: 2012). These are normal parameters by which the child's growth and development are assessed.

Development refers to an increase in complexity of function and progression of skills. These are qualitative changes that define the child as a unique individual. As the child grows, maturity progresses and function becomes more defined. For example, a 3-month-old child, unlike a month-old child, is expected to hold its head firm and follow objects with its eyes without turning the head; yet children at both ages (1 month and 3 months) respond to discomfort or attract attention by crying. This action of crying becomes differentiated with development. For example, at 3 months the child employs the whole body to cry, whereby the face is contorted, there are tears flowing, arms thrash and legs kick in the air. At 9 months, only the contorted face and tears denote crying and the thrashing and kicking of legs may be explained as 'tantrums'.

Growth and development are integrated and interlinked from head to toe (cephalo-caudal). Each body system runs to its own growth and development schedule, with the nervous, cardiovascular and respiratory systems taking the lead well ahead of the other systems, such as the immune and reproductive systems. Progression is also marked by increased integration of growth, development and the environment, indicating maturity, where the sequence of physical changes is related to genetic factors (internal environment) and influenced by external environmental factors. For example, holding the body upright starts with the head, then the back muscles that allow the child to sit, then the lower limbs that allow the child to stand. Behaviour also becomes sophisticated with incremental skill development. This depends on nerve myelination and stimulation, whereby a highly stimulated child is able to achieve milestones much earlier than a child with less or no stimulation.

Factors that influence growth and development in child care

From conception, child growth and development is a delicate process that requires collaboration for it to be successful. During pregnancy, the mother has to be healthy so that she can provide a healthy and supportive internal environment for the child, hence the early attendance to antenatal care. At birth, the newborn has to be assisted to adapt to the external environment. Adaptation is a term that refers to the child's body's adjustment and accommodation to environmental factors, such as the temperature, light, hygiene, nutrition, elimination, comfort and discomfort.

The child's growth and development pattern is characteristic but unique for every child. This includes rapid growth in the first year, slow growth during middle and late childhood, losing primary teeth during middle childhood, and the appearance of secondary sex characteristics during early adolescence. This is influenced by:

Family. The family is by far the most important determinant of who we are. The family provides for both the internal and external environments.
- *Heredity*. The genes that each person acquires from the parents determine what that person will look like, sex, height, weight, and in some instances the health.

- *Socioeconomic environment.* The family will again play a role in the value system, customs, traditions, social, economic, emotional climate and provision of resources. As children grow they are socialised into familial and societal norms.

Community. As the child grows, there is extension of association into the community, society, school and religion. Activities such as play and attending school are very significant in making the child a functioning member of society – someone who can relate to others, share, appreciate and be considerate. The community helps in shaping the child's interactions.

Health. The health of both the mother and the child determines the child's growth and ability to function. From conception, the mother has to be healthy, hence the antenatal care, where all impediments are identified, be it nutrition or health of the mother. A healthy child is much more likely to follow the normal pattern of growth and development than a child with ill health. The causes of ill health can be congenital, where there are health-limiting congenital, mechanical or chemical defects, such as transposition of great vessels or congenital hypothyroidism. These may require surgical or medical management.

Normal milestones in a child's development

Milestones are steps or stages that are followed in growth and development. They are observable and measurable in quantity (days, weeks, months and years) and quality. Milestones include functions such as responses as indicated in the reflexes, eg the startle reflex when frightened (see Table 1.1).

Table 1.1 Developmental milestones

Age	Gross motor	Fine motor	Speech/ language	Cognitive/ problem solving	Social emotions
1 month	• Primitive reflexes: moro, startle, flexor	• Primitive reflexes: firm grasp	• Primitive responses: rooting, sucking, swallowing, crying, startles to loud noises	• Tends to fix gaze, usually on mother's face and follow objects slowly to midline • Startles with high-pitched sounds	• Responds to soothing cuddles/ touch
2 months	• Head steady momentarily when held up • Raises head up 45° in a prone position	• Fingers flexed	• Coos, turns face to voice	• Follows objects past midline	• Presents a social smile when stroked under the chin

Age	Gross motor	Fine motor	Speech/language	Cognitive/problem solving	Social emotions
4 months	• Sits with support • Raises head up 90° in prone position	• Palmar grasp Can hold a rattle and shake it • Reaches out to obtain items • Brings objects to midline	• Laughs, squeals, monosyllables	• Anticipates routine • Prefers usual caregiver • Purposeful exploration of objects using eyes, hands, mouth	• Explores parents'/caregivers' faces • Communicates with parent/caregiver • Responds to parents' voices
6 months	• Sits with minimal support and falls forward on hands • Rolls side-to-side • Head steady	• Transfers objects from hand to hand • Grasp clumsy • Brings objects to mouth	• Head turns to respond to noise • Babbles nonspecific sounds	• Follows objects from side to side, up and down • Looks for dropped or partially hidden objects • Aware of strangers and expresses anxiety over strangers	• Expresses emotions: happiness, sadness, anger • Holds out arms to be picked up
9 months	• Sitting without support • Pulls self to a standing position • Creeps on hands and knees (crawls)	• Inferior pincer grip • Pokes at objects	• Initiates sounds • Able to say 'mama', 'dada' and show gestures indicating 'bye-bye' by waving a hand	• Uncovers toys, plays 'Peek-a-boo' • Follows objects in all directions • Follows a rolling ball	• Establishes relationships • Demonstrates separation anxiety • Helps with dressing, feeds self and chews
12 months	• Stands unassisted. • Wide-based gait and walks a few steps.	• Fine pincer grip replaces palmar grasp. • Finger-feeds self. • Throws objects.	• May say one word with meaning (eg 'no') • Responds to own name. • Follows 1-step commands with gestures.	• Uses objects functionally, eg rolls toy cars. • Initiates gestures and sounds.	• Points at wanted items. • Narrative memory begins.

Age	Gross motor	Fine motor	Speech/language	Cognitive/problem solving	Social emotions
15 months	• Walks well	• Uses a spoon, can open a bottle top, can build a tower of 2 blocks	• Points to 1 body part • Knows at least 5 words of jargon • Can follow 1-step command with no gestures	• Experiments with toys to make them work	• Points at interesting items to share and experience • Can fetch and bring to caregiver
18 months	• Stoops and recovers • Runs	• Carries toys while walking • Removes clothing • Can build a tower of 4 blocks • Fisted pencil grip to start scribbling	• Points to 3 body parts • Knows 10 to 25 words • Labels familiar objects	• Symbolic play with doll or teddy bear, eg 'give teddy a drink'	• Increased independence, parallel play
2 years	• Jumps on two feet • Goes up and down stairs	• Uses a fork to feed self • Can build a tower of 6 blocks	• 50+ words • Able to use plurals correctly eg 'I', 'me', 'you', 'me and', 'we' • Can follow a 2-step command	• Searches for hidden objects after multiple replacements	• Can throw tantrums to indicate disagreement and says 'no' • Demonstrates possessiveness: 'mine'
3 years	• Can climb up the stairs	• Undresses • Potty trained • Draws circles and turns pages of a book	• Can follow a 3-step command • Knows about 200 words Is about 75% intelligible • Can pose questions like 'why' • Can state full name, age and gender	• Understands simple time concepts • Identifies shapes • Compares 2 items for size • Counts up to 3	• Roleplay, cooperative play, sharing • Understands that separation is not permanent

Age	Gross motor	Fine motor	Speech/ language	Cognitive/ problem solving	Social emotions
4 years	• Hops on 1 foot • Can walk down the stairs	• Can cut shapes with scissors • Can cut buttons with a pair of scissors • Can write 'x' and draw a square	• Sentences are 100% intelligible • Can tell a story • Applies correct tenses	• Counts up to 4 • Can identify up to 4 colours • Can identify opposite, eg black and white	• Has preferred friends • Fantasy play
5 years	• Can balance on 1 foot • Can skip • Can ride a bicycle (if available)	• Can point at and identify 10 body parts • Tripod pencil grasp • Can write own name • Can wash, dress, and feed self, including tying shoe laces	• All tenses 100% (present, past, future) • Talking intelligibly with >5000 words Is able to make jokes	• Counts to 10 accurately • Recites alphabet by rote learning • Recognises some letters	• Has a group of friends • Follows group rules • Games have rules and these are followed

Conclusion

The growth and development of a child may, in many instances, be a marvel to the parents. Children in their uniqueness achieve their milestones differently. A healthy child who is stimulated will move from one stage of development to the other with much ease, unlike a child that lacks stimulation and may struggle with progress in their growth and development. Relationships with children should bear their developmental stage in mind, as these relationships may help or hinder development; the relationships themselves may be influenced by the specific child's stage of development.

Suggested activities for learners

Activity 1.1
1. In a maximum of 10 lines, integrate and explain growth and development in child care.
   (In your explanation, use the words growth, development, maturation, cephalo-caudal, proximo-distal.)
2. Describe the factors that influence growth and development in child care.

References

Harrison, V. 2012. *The newborn baby*. 6th edition. Cape Town: Juta.

Hockenberry, MJ & Wilson, D. 2015. *Wong's nursing care of infants and children*. 10th edition. Elsevier.

Mogotlane, S, Mokoena, J, Chauke, M, Matlakala, M, Young, A & Randa, B. 2018. *Juta's complete textbook of medical surgical nursing*. 2nd edition. Cape Town: Juta.

Mott, SR, James, SR & Sperhac AM. 1990. *Nursing care of children and families*. 2nd edition. New York: Addison-Wesley Nursing.

2 Reactions of a child to hospitalisation

LEARNING OBJECTIVES

At the end of this Chapter, you should be able to:
- explain the behaviour displayed by hospitalised children
- assess the needs of hospitalised children and the support their parents and siblings require
- effectively plan, implement and evaluate the physical, emotional and psychological care provided to hospitalised children and their families in order to help them cope with separation and speedy recovery from surgery.

KEY CONCEPTS AND TERMINOLOGY

family:	A social unit where people are in a relationship and provide physical, emotional, psychological and economical support to each other.
informed consent:	Permission granted to perform a procedure or provide treatment after a full explanation of and information about the said procedure/treatment has been given.
hospitalisation:	A term used to describe an act of keeping sick people in hospital for the purposes of medical and/or surgical treatment.
separation:	This is an act where the child is kept away from those he knows and derives comfort from.
siblings:	Biological relatives (sisters and brothers) in a family unit.

PREREQUISITE KNOWLEDGE
- Anatomy and physiology of the human body
- Applied social sciences.

MEDICO-LEGAL CONSIDERATIONS

Child care is risk laden. Children are prone to accidents and mishaps. All injuries sustained by the child/patient while in the hospital are regarded as a serious adverse event (SAE). The family may litigate and the hospital may have to bear the consequences, therefore it is imperative to ensure safety of all children when hospitalised. An example of an SAE is when children in hospital are cared for in unusually high cot beds and could fall if the cot sides are not closed. They can pick up needles and blades and prick or cut themselves. So even before the surgical procedures, mechanical injuries are possible. Because of the small size and lack of maturity of the patient, it is important for the medical team to exercise extra care in calculating doses of medications to be administered to avoid an overdose, as well as in choosing instruments to use on the child because of the smaller size of their body structures, eg nasogastric tubes, tracheostomy tubes. Procedures have to be explained carefully to parents/guardians for them to give the necessary consent and to communicate to them that the Minister of Health, through the chief/clinical executive officer (CEO) of the hospital, has a right to give consent for treatment should he deem it fit to save the life of a child.

ETHICAL CONSIDERATIONS

When children are hospitalised, they may be separated from their families. This separation can be traumatic to a child, regardless of age. The separation may be worse in cases where surgery is to be performed as, added to the fear of separation, there may be the fear of painful injections, surgical cuts, blood and the unknown. If it is planned surgery and the child is old enough to be engaged in a conversation, explain to the child why they are in hospital and have to be left in hospital; why injections have to be given; and why they may see blood on the dressings. It is also advisable to explain activities like injections, dressings and the administration of oral medications. Where possible, ask the child for permission to perform these activities. The Children's Act of 2005 specifies that a child may consent to medical treatment, surgical operations, HIV testing, decision on the disclosure of their HIV status from the age of 12 with specific provisions (Children's Act 38 of 2005, Sections 129, 130, 131,132, 133, 134 and 142). In South Africa, the common-law requirement for consent is that it must be given by a person capable in law to do so. The person giving the consent must be informed, the information must be specific, address one issue and one issue only, and the information must be clear and unambiguous.

ESSENTIAL HEALTH LITERACY

It is important to explain to parents/guardians the process to be followed when surgery is to be performed, starting from the admission of the child and what this means for and to them and the child. The separation that will happen needs to be understood from the beginning. The operation that is to be performed has to be explained in detail to get the parents' support, as this may assist in putting the child at ease. It is also necessary to get the guardians to sign the consent form, stating that they understand the operation that is to be performed, its benefits and its risks. It is at this point that parents are assured that the child will only be discharged when they can manage the wound and the child is out of danger.

Introduction

Much like the first day of school, illness and hospitalisation can be one of the first life crises children experience because of the separation which is almost always inevitable if the child is to be hospitalised. Without separation, children have a tremendous capacity to withstand stress. When hospitalised, the child has to be admitted into the hospital, with some hospitals requiring parents to leave the child behind with strangers in a strange environment. This is made worse by the painful treatments that can be interpreted as bodily harm by children, and the manner in which nursing interventions are carried out. Furthermore, a hospitalised child loses some measure of control and has to depend on other people to manage their environment. They now have to follow the hospital routine and abandon the routine that they are used to in their home environment. These experiences may evoke feelings of guilt in a child who might consider hospitalisation as punishment for some wrongdoing.

Some hospitals have a policy that allows mothers to lodge with the child, depending on the age of the child. This always makes hospital stay much more acceptable to the child.

Reaction of a child to hospitalisation

The reactions to hospitalisation may vary and are influenced by the age of the child, previous separation from parents/guardians, previous experience with illness, the seriousness of the diagnosis, acquired coping skills, the reaction of the parents/guardians to the child's illness, and other support systems available to the child and the parents/guardians. Children's reaction to stress is predictable and is explained in three stages:

Protest. When children are faced with a threatening situation, they may become anxious and afraid. This may be expressed by loud screams and aggression. The child may hold on to the parent/guardian, cling and cry even louder when the parent/guardian is about to leave them. As the parent continues to leave, they may even run after the parent and may attack the care team with fists, bites and kicks if these try to stop them. Afterwards, when the parents are gone, the child may even try to escape from the scene in search of the parents, hence the reason why children's wards are always closed with secure access and, sometimes, security guards at the ward entrance.

> **Clinical alert!**
> A healthy protest persists every time the parent visits and leaves.

The management of this stage includes:
- frequent visits from parents and siblings, until the child understands that they are not being abandoned but it is necessary for them to be in hospital to be well and be discharged home. At this stage, the family itself needs much understanding and support from the care team. They must not be criticised for the child's behaviour, which must never be interpreted as 'unruly', 'spoilt', 'attention seeking' or any nasty comments.

Despair. If the parent does not make any appearance, or does not visit or visits are infrequent, the child may interpret their protest to have failed and the parent to have abandoned them. The crying will stop, the child will be withdrawn, activity decreases, there is lack of interest in surroundings, play and food, and the child becomes visibly depressed. This is the stage of despair. The child gives up the fight for the parent to stay with them or return to stay. At this stage, the child may regress to earlier behaviour such as crawling while already walking, bed-wetting, baby talk or becoming quiet and uncommunicative.

> **Clinical alert!**
> A healthy state of affairs is for the child to return to the protest stage should the parent visit. The parents must be encouraged to visit regardless of the return to the protest staged by the child each time they visit.

The stage of despair is managed by encouraging the family to visit frequently and not allow the child to miss them and be depressed. A favourite toy, blanket or 'object of security' may be kept with the child, if allowed. This object keeps the child feeling connected to their family and home as it may carry the usual smells of the child's environment back home. The nurses must not deny the child contact with this object.

Should the parents take too long to visit, the child may then go into a depression as explained above.

Detachment or denial: At this stage, it may appear as though the child has come to terms with the separation. This is when the protests and the depression have not resulted in the parents coming to visit or stay. The child becomes cooperative, plays amicably with others and interacts better with strangers, who, in this case, are the caregivers. This is false acceptance of the loss the child is suffering. It might cause lifelong scars that will manifest in a range of negative behaviours, such as mistrust of adults, hatred, unresolved anger and revenge.

Reaction of parents to the child's hospitalisation

Childhood illness and hospitalisation are often unpleasant for the family. The reaction of parents is influenced by a variety of factors: the events leading to the child's illness, the seriousness of the diagnosis and the current condition of the child. Other factors may include cultural and belief system, the support that parents have in the family, as well as current tensions in the family. Parents may be fearful of the outcome of hospitalisation and therefore try to cope with uncertainty. They may take their desperation and despair out on the care team, demanding some explanation of the child's diagnosis in the hope of learning something positive each time. They may feel helpless, and may start to question the adequacy of the facility and the competence of the care staff. They may also have feelings of guilt or believe that the injury or illness is a result of their negligence.

The reactions of parents are managed through the provision of information. The reactions they exhibit are usually as a result of fear of the unknown. Information about the child's illness must be provided unreservedly, about what will happen, who is going to do what, when and how to contact the ward and the various people who will provide the required information. Information about the hospital routine and rules must be given – what is allowed and what is not allowed and why. The information given to the parents will assist them in handling siblings, relatives and friends. If required, a psychologist must be consulted to assist them to cope with the situation. The nurse must establish a trusting relationship with the parents, listen to their concerns, acknowledge their feelings and support them unconditionally.

Reaction of siblings to hospitalisation

The reaction of siblings is usually a mixture of feelings and emotions such as loneliness, anxiety, fear, worry, even anger, resentment, jealousy and guilt. The siblings may miss the hospitalised child when sharing their daily activities and may be angry at the illness that has caused this separation. In some instances, siblings might be angry with the parents for paying more attention to the hospitalised child, or compromising their care at home. The siblings are sometimes jealous of their sick brother or sister, as the sick child, in their reckoning, is receiving better care than they are, with parents having to spend time in hospital or having to leave the other siblings with neighbours or relatives. The siblings may suffer guilt, thinking that their actions might have caused the illness, for example, in the case of a fracture sustained during play. Furthermore, children may fear death of their sibling, especially if they know someone who died in hospital.

Management of siblings
Hospitalisation of a sibling can cause psychological harm to those left at home. It is important that everybody in the family is aware of the need for hospitalisation for the child. If possible, the remaining siblings must be informed about the pending hospitalisation. They must be involved in the preparation of the child and in becoming familiar with things like the purpose of the hospital, what the inside of the hospital looks like, the activities that go on in the hospital, the ward, the hospital bed, the nurses, doctors and other health workers, including the cleaners. The siblings must understand the reason why their brother or sister has to be in hospital so that they may get help which is not available at home. No one must be made to feel guilty or responsible for the hospitalisation. The diagnosis and its prognosis must be explained in the most positive manner without raising undue hope where there is none. If they are to be left behind when parents go to the hospital to visit, arrangements with a carer, neighbours or relatives must be made in consultation with them. Time must be allowed for them to visit the hospital to see their sibling. Ensure that their excitement does not exhaust the sick child, but the visit must be memorable and all must look forward to the next visit.

Bringing food into hospital

Hospitals have a legal obligation to comply with the requirements of the Food Safety Act of 1990 and associated legislation relating to the composition, labelling, safety, handling, control and hygiene of food. Hospitals may develop standard operating procedures (SOPs) relating to food and paediatric wards. Any food brought in should be suitable for the dietary needs of the patient. Visitors should be encouraged to bring patients food that contributes to a healthy, balanced diet. Any advice regarding the suitability of foods can be obtained from the nurse in charge or dietician. On arrival at the ward, all food gifts should be declared. A trained nurse will check to see if the food is suitable for the patient and check containers and labelling. Patients on 'nil per os' should be kept separate from those who can eat to avoid delay of operations.

Assessment and common findings
Subjective data
There is a lot that the nurses must know about the child on admission for them to be able to help the child cope with hospitalisation. Although most of the conversation is with the adults, the child must not be excluded from the interview, by periodically paying attention through play and occasionally directing some questions to the child to try to establish rapport. The adult who is with the child must give information about the child's health problem, its presentation, duration, types of treatments tried, where and by whom. It is also important to give a family history to exclude hereditary factors. The nurse will also

need to know the child's routine, habits such as sleeping time, elimination, meals, day naps, and any 'objects of security' that the child depends on, such as a blanket, a doll, teddy bear or soft toy.

Objective data

The physical examination is the child's first contact with healthcare staff. Activities such as the recording of the vital signs, weight, height, head circumference and skin condition should be done. The assistance of the parents may be needed to achieve the results successfully. Other activities such as blood and radiological tests might be the child's first encounter with pain and distress.

Assisting the child to adapt in hospital
The role of parents

The role of parents is to provide for physical and emotional care, supporting and encouraging the child throughout hospitalisation. In some hospitals parents are allowed to stay in hospital with the child, in line with the hospital's policy. The nurse has to assess family needs to allow them to carry out their care tasks. The parents also get a chance to practise care under supervision.

> **Practice alert!**
>
> It is important to make the child comfortable from the beginning. You can achieve this by continuing to talk to the family and allow the child to observe from a safe distance. For instance, if the child has a doll, initiate a conversation about the doll, such as, 'Does your doll have a name?', 'Where does your doll live?'. This might draw the child into the conversation.

Steps to assist the child in coping with hospitalisation

- Encourage parental involvement in the care of the child. Parents and/or guardians should be offered accommodation in the hospital or ward where possible. Neonates, very sick children and adolescents need their parents to be around them when stressed.
- Whenever possible, parents should arrange for special leave at their workplaces so that they can be with their children. Many constitutions recognise child illness as a family responsibility.
- Assist parents in obtaining information concerning the condition of the child and the treatment plan; explain all procedures.
- Orientate the family to the hospital routine and explain the ward routine and rules.
- Offer temporary assistance for the parents to have a break in the care of their child.
- Reinforce positive parenting, such as body contact.

Sibling participation

It is important to identify the needs of siblings and help the parents in meeting these while looking after their sick child. This is done by:
- keeping siblings informed about the child's illness and progress thereof
- allowing siblings to visit the hospitalised child in line with the hospital or ward's visitation rules
- allowing the older siblings to assist in the care of the sick child if they so wish.

Information for visiting siblings

1. Siblings have to be informed about why they have to wash their hands before and after touching the sick brother or sister.
2. Sick siblings are not allowed to visit.
3. Depending on each hospital's policies, children who are not siblings of the patient may not be allowed to visit.

Child's participation in own care

Children need information about themselves to be able to take an interest in their care. Depending on the child's age and understanding, it is important that the child is told about their illness, the proposed treatment and care so that they can express their views if they so wish. This shows respect and, by so doing, the child is empowered and gains control of the environment in which they find themselves. More than anything, the child needs to establish a trusting relationship with the nurses. So, they need to be informed about every event and encouraged to express their feelings and anxieties about the event.

Methods of communicating information to the child

These vary depending on age and maturity. It could be through:
- storytelling or reading a story book
- pictures, videos and slides
- puppet shows
- play – either playing with toys or through roleplay
- safe and supervised handling of medical equipment.

Pain in children

Pain and painful treatments are one of the major reasons for fear of hospitalisation. Previously it was thought that infants did not feel pain because of an immature nervous system in which the nerves were not completely myelinated. Nowadays there is little doubt that infants feel pain, or more specifically, react to obnoxious stimuli with distress indicative of pain.

Children fear pain and unfortunately nurses may underestimate and undertreat pain in children. One of the reasons for inadequate management of pain is a lack of understanding of what pain is, because it is subjective and children have difficulty communicating the pain they experience. An operational definition of pain by the International Association of Study of Pain (IASP) is: 'an unpleasant sensory and emotional experience associated with actual or potential tissue damage' (Kumar and Elavarasi, 2016).

Principles of pain assessment in children

To assess pain, do the following:
- ask the child about pain
- ask the parents about pain

- use pain rating scales
- evaluate behavioural changes
- evaluate physiological changes.

Questioning the child about pain
It is difficult to elicit the definition of pain from a child, because in some instances the child might not know the meaning of pain or the child might deny pain from fear of injectable medication to treat pain. The child can be asked to locate pain or to describe the feeling in his or her own words. Questions asked include:
- Tell me about the hurt you have.
- What do you do when you hurt?
- What do you want others to do for you when you hurt?
- What helps the most to take away your hurt?
- Is there something special that you want me to know about you when you hurt?

Questioning parents about the child's pain
Parents are the main source of information, as they know the child best and are in a better position to notice behaviour changes. They also need to realise that their knowledge of their child is important in providing quality care. Questions about the child's pain include the following:
- Describe to me the pain your child is experiencing.
- How does your child react to pain?
- Does your child tell you when they are hurting?
- How do you know when your child is hurting?
- What do you do to ease discomfort for your child when your child is hurting?
- What does your child do to get relief when hurting?
- Which of these actions work best to decrease or take away your child's hurt?
- Is there something special that you want me to know about your child and their pain?

Pain rating scales
- There are several measures that can be used to analyse the intensity of pain in children. Most of these can be described within the child's behavior and facial expression. The Faces Scale is one of the methods that can be used to rate the degree or intensity of pain in children. The scale consists of 6 cartoon faces from a smiling face for no pain to a tearful face for severe pain.

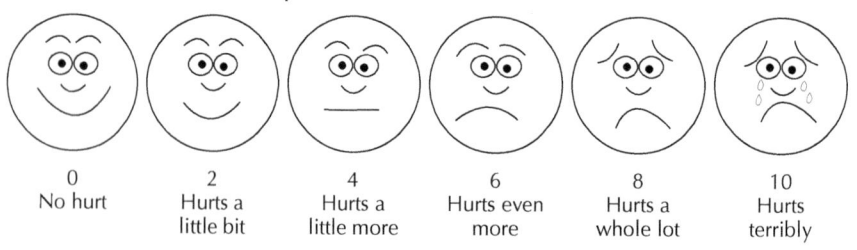

0	2	4	6	8	10
No hurt	Hurts a little bit	Hurts a little more	Hurts even more	Hurts a whole lot	Hurts terribly

Responses when in pain
Behavioural changes
Behavioural changes are important in assessing pain in non-verbal individuals like children, for example the rubbing of eyes or pulling of ears if these are sore.

Physiological changes
Physiological changes indicative of pain include flushing or pallor of the skin, sweating, an increase in the pulse rate, respiration and blood pressure, restlessness and dilatation of the pupils.

Conclusion
The management of the child's, parents' and siblings' reaction to hospitalisation includes provision of information. Children, especially the very young, may imagine things and fantasise and this can create a lot of anxiety, uncertainty, fear and worry. Therefore, it is important to communicate the situation to the child in a manner that they will understand. This may involve showing the child photographs of the hospital, allowing them to walk around the ward so that they are aware of their surroundings, allowing them to calmly touch the hospital bed and medical equipment that is not dangerous for them to handle. Siblings must be provided with information and explanations of what is happening in the hospital to the brother or sister. Where possible, they must be allowed to visit the hospitalised sibling and, if possible, allowed to talk and touch them and their bandages. This will help dissipate the myth of hospitalisation. If siblings are not able to visit the hospital, proper arrangements to care for the remaining siblings must be made in consultation with them. They should never feel neglected or left with strangers without prior consultation with them.

Suggested activities for learners

Activity 2.1
1. Describe behaviour that would be considered healthy in a child who is hospitalised.
2. Explain the preparation that should be done to ensure that children cope with hospitalisation.

References
Harrison, V. 2012. *The newborn baby*. 6th edition. Cape Town: Juta.
Hockenberry, MJ & Wilson, D. 2015. *Wong's nursing care of infants and children*. 10th edition. Elsevier.
Mogotlane, S, Mokoena, J, Chauke, M, Matlakala, M, Young, A & Randa, B. 2018. *Juta's complete textbook of medical surgical nursing*. 2nd edition. Cape Town: Juta.
Mott, SR, James, SR & Sperhac, AM. 1990. *Nursing care of children and families*. 2nd edition. New York: Addison-Wesley Nursing.

Section 2

Introduction to surgical nursing in child care

3 Nursing care of a child in the pre-operative period

LEARNING OBJECTIVES

On completion of this Chapter, you should be able to:
- describe the specific needs of a child who is to undergo surgery
- explain the principles of surgical nursing in child care
- explain pre-operative assessment findings and interpret diagnostic tests that are related to the facilitation of recovery from surgery
- describe specific pre-operative nursing interventions to facilitate the child's recovery from surgery
- discuss the importance of a valid consent
- provide essential health information to the child and their parents or guardians to alleviate fear and anxiety related to surgery.

KEY CONCEPTS AND TERMINOLOGY	
assent:	Refers to affirmative agreement of a minor who is to take part in the informed-consent procedure in a way adapted to his or her capabilities, while the legal representative has the formal role of consenting.
informed consent:	The patient's (child's) decision to agree to undergo surgery and/or the parents'/guardians' decision to agree that the child should undergo surgery, following a thorough explanation of the surgical procedure and a complete understanding of the information provided by the surgeon thereof, the reasons for the surgical procedure, the benefits and the risks involved.
intraoperative care:	This is care that is given to a patient from the time they are transferred to the operating table until the operation is completed and they are returned to the recovery room.
perioperative nursing care:	Nursing interventions during the pre-operative, intraoperative and postoperative periods.
postoperative care:	Nursing interventions rendered to the patient after surgery from the time the patient is transferred from the recovery room to the surgical ward or intensive care unit until discharge, inclusive of follow-up visits.

premedication:	Medication prescribed for patients to calm them down and pre-empt anaesthesia before undergoing surgery.
postoperative medication:	Medication prescribed for patients to assist in their post-operative recovery, pain management and care.
pre-operative care:	Nursing interventions to help the patient keep calm, alleviate fear and anxiety related to surgery to facilitate recovery post-surgery. Pre-operative care commences from the time a decision to operate on a patient is taken and lasts up to the time the patient arrives in the operating theatre or room for surgery.

PREREQUISITE KNOWLEDGE

- Human anatomy and physiology
- Pharmacology
- Biochemistry and biophysics as applied to nursing care
- Microbiology and parasitology
- Application of universal precautions regarding infection control
- Applied social sciences and communication
- Family and community health as it applies to child care
- Professional, ethical and legal framework of nursing in South Africa
- Principles of record-keeping.

MEDICO-LEGAL CONSIDERATIONS

Nursing care of children to undergo surgery is a risk-laden exercise, which demands thorough assessment of patients, failure of which can result in mismanagement of conditions and litigation. The nurse must therefore assess the child comprehensively and keep a complete and accurate record of all assessments (subjective and objective) done. The age, weight and health status are particularly important for the calculation of medications, fluids, electrolyte, etc.

ETHICAL CONSIDERATIONS

The attending surgeon has a responsibility to provide the parents and, in some instances, the child, with full information about the operation so that the consent that the surgeon obtains and guardians sign is based on information and understanding (informed consent). It is important for nurses to keep the information about the surgical procedure, its nature and extent confidential, disclosure of which has to be with permission from the relevant principals. In accordance with the Constitution of the Republic of South Africa and the South African Patient's Rights Charter, parents and, in some instances, the child must be allowed to exercise their right to participate in their child's/own care and decision making. For example, in a case where the parents are refusing to give consent for a life-saving procedure (such as a blood transfusion required for a child from a Jehovah's Witness family) the Children's Act allows the Minister of Health, through the chief executive officer of the hospital, to supersede the decision of the parents.

ESSENTIAL HEALTH LITERACY

Parents or guardians of children to undergo surgery are usually anxious about the surgery and its outcome. They are anxious about the separation from and hospitalisation of their child. They may be worried about the outcomes of the surgery, how the child will cope with hospitalisation, separation and the surgery. The child is usually anxious about separation from the family, hospitalisation, anaesthesia, and painful procedures and treatments. Communication becomes one of the most important tools to manage these aspects. The parent and the child must be provided with information on what hospitalisation and the operation entail and how challenges will be addressed. For planned surgery, the child must be allowed pre-operative visits to familiarise him- or herself with the hospital environment and, where possible, the operating theatre, to be shown on a video without trivialising the seriousness of the business of the operating room, the intensive care unit as well as the high care and the general surgical care units. During these pre-operative visits it is important for parents and the child to understand the positive and the negative aspects of the procedure and the hospitalisation.

Introduction

Surgery is an important treatment option in the management of childhood conditions. It is done to correct and repair congenital defects, repair acquired injuries such as fractures, remove defective tissue, make diagnosis from biopsy and cure conditions such as abscesses. Surgery, be it elective or an emergency, continues to be a strange experience, especially for the child and the family. It involves psychosocial, emotional, spiritual and physical dimensions. Certain legal and ethical prescriptions must be taken into account, for example, the signing of an informed consent based on provision of complete information about the surgery to be performed, the reason for the surgery, the names of the surgeon/s involved, possible outcomes of the surgery, and prognosis postoperatively. Parents need to be given time to think about whether they will agree to the operation or not and should not be coerced into signing the consent form. The nurse has the responsibility to provide a safe, therapeutic and caring environment for the child, reassuring the family on positive outcomes based on previous experiences. Care must be taken not to raise expectations of relatives especially on positive outcomes because surgery, no matter how minor, carries risks.

> **Clinical alert!**
> Advances in medicine are slowly rendering surgery redundant. Many inflammatory conditions, including abscesses that would previously require surgical management, are no longer surgical problems because of the effective antibiotics available in the market. Surgery, where possible, is avoided, except for correction of congenital defects, and repair of torn or wasted tissues, including fractures and correction for function.

Indications for surgery

The following are indications for surgery:
- Congenital defects which, at birth, are life-threatening, such as oesophageal atresia with or without tracheal fistula, and transposition of the great blood vessels
- Congenital defects which need repair for improved quality of life, such as the cleft lip and palate
- Acquired defects for which medical management is not appropriate, such as intussusception, volvulus, fractures or tumours
- To establish or confirm a diagnosis, for example, the removal and examination of suspicious tissue to determine pathology (biopsy) or the extent thereof and various exploratory procedures.

Suffixes used to describe surgical procedures

A suffix is a descriptive term at the end of a stem word. For example '-ectomy' is to remove.
- **ectomy:** removal of a body part, eg appendicectomy (removal of the appendix)
- **orrhaphy:** repair of a body structure, eg herniorrhaphy (repair of a hernia, which is done when an organ is prolapsing through a weakened area of the muscular wall)
- **oscopy:** looking into a hollow organ using a scope, eg bronchoscopy (looking into the bronchi), where anaesthesia may be necessary to relax the patient
- **ostomy:** cutting an opening into a hollow organ, eg tracheostomy (opening into the trachea)
- **otomy:** creation of an opening into a body structure, eg craniotomy (opening into the cranium or skull)
- **plasty:** reconstruction or repair of an area of the body, eg tympanoplasty (repair of the tympanic membrane of the ear).

Classification and types of surgery

There is more than one way to classify surgery, as shown in Table 3.1 below.

Table 3.1 Classification of surgery

Classification	Types of surgery
According to the extent of the procedure, the possible effects on the body, and the known risks of the procedure	**Minor surgery.** In children there is no minor surgery, but for clarity minor surgery can be regarded as that which causes relatively little disruption of function and has few risks. **Major surgery.** The procedure may cause considerable disruption of function and the risks involved are greater. Surgery that involves the opening of any body cavity is always classified as a major procedure, eg repair of the diaphragmatic hernia.

According to the objective and the character of the procedure	**Ablative surgery.** The total removal of a diseased organ or structure, for example the removal of cancerous organs and tissues. **Constructive/corrective surgery.** The correction of abnormal anatomy to improve function, for example, the reconstruction of the rectum and anus in anorectal malformations. **Cosmetic surgery.** The repair of parts of the body to improve appearance as perceived by the patient, for example, a cleft lip and palate. **Curative surgery.** Performed in order to arrest a pathological process, such as the Ramstedt operation in hypertrophied pyloric stenosis. **Palliative or non-curative surgery.** Performed to alleviate symptoms and improve the quality of life of the patient, eg cerebrospinal fluid drainage pipe to relieve intracranial pressure. **Diagnostic surgery.** Carried out in order to establish a diagnosis, for example, a biopsy. **Exploratory surgery.** Carried out to assess the extent of a lesion or pathology. **Prophylactic surgery.** The removal of tissue and/or organs that are not vital and are likely to develop into a disease, for example, polyps. **Reconstructive surgery.** Performed to reconstruct a defect or in response to trauma in an attempt to improve function, to obtain a more desirable cosmetic effect or to restore normal appearance, for example, plastic surgery for burn wounds.
According to the urgency of the procedure	**Elective surgery.** This is planned and scheduled at the convenience of both the patient and the surgeon. Elective surgery involves conditions where the patient's pathology can be controlled until conditions are favourable for surgery, or where the patient is neither endangered nor seriously inconvenienced if surgery is postponed, eg the cleft lip and palate is done when the child is at least 3 months old. **Emergency surgery.** This is urgent and must be performed as soon as possible, often immediately. This type of surgery is necessary in life-threatening conditions, eg oesophageal atresia with or without tracheal fistula.

The needs of a child who is to undergo surgery

The child who is to undergo surgery has specific needs which the nurse must assist with:
Nutrition and fluid intake. A child going for surgery needs to be starved overnight to avoid aspiration during anaesthesia. At the same time children cannot go without fluids for extended periods and need fluids for positive outcomes post-surgery. Whereas solids

could be withheld for 6 hours, fluids should only be withheld for 4 hours. An intravenous infusion is put up 6 hours prior to the operation so that when oral intake is withheld, the child's hydration is maintained. A strict record of the fluid run intake through the IV therapy, and subsequent output, is kept to avoid over- or underhydration. This is measured against the output of all kinds, ie wet nappies, stools passed, amount and consistency, insensible loss, etc.

Warmth. The child must be kept warm by adequate cover, but not hot. Avoid artificial warming with electric blankets, except in the case of a neonate who should be kept in the incubator at all times. Avoid visible sweating.

Skin preparation. The child must be bathed and dressed in clean clothes, nappy changed and comfortable. Ensure that the skin integrity is maintained. Any potential septic foci should be treated and cleared prior to surgery. Hair must be shaved, if necessary, to clear the operation site.

Rest and sleep. The nurse should make sure that the patient is comfortable and is not unduly disturbed during the night. A sedative may be prescribed as part of the patient's premedication.

Safety and patient identification. Ensure that the patient is adequately identified in line with their patient's file, by name and surname, hospital admission registration number, ward where admitted, proposed surgical procedure, name of surgeon responsible and date of operation. These details are also to be reflected on the name tag around the wrist or ankle. Another identity tag with a different colour may be used to indicate any added medical conditions, such as hypertension/diabetes mellitus. Another safety measure relates to precautions that are taken to ensure that the child does not eat or drink 2 to 4 hours before surgery. 'Nil per os' signs must be displayed on the child's bed and guardians and visitors must be cautioned on the meaning of the sign. This is very important in children as they may not be able to talk for themselves or help you in this regard, and it ensures safety.

Site marking. Site marking is a form of identification where the site to be operated upon must be marked with an indelible marker on the body, and written in bold in the patient's file. This is to prevent mistakes in operating the wrong site or limb, as the case might be.

Psychological care and comfort. Children, regardless of age, are sensitive to any change in the environment or routine and must therefore be psychologically prepared for the forthcoming experience. The parent/guardian must be allowed to stay with the child, touch and talk to them, even if the child is under sedation. Crying must be minimised. Activities and procedures are to be explained to the parent/guardian and child to alleviate anxiety about both. Encourage the parent/guardian to participate in the care of the child. Give the name and an explanation of the procedure to be done, the purpose, the premedication, anaesthesia, duration of the procedure and anticipated outcomes and even adverse effects without scaring them.

Nursing assessment and common findings in a patient to undergo surgery

A full assessment of the child will be done by the nurse, the surgeon, the aneasthetist and, where possible, the theatre nurse. The purpose of such an assessment is to identify factors that might impact on the course and outcome of surgery.

Clinical alert!

Patients' perioperative documents must demonstrate that safety checks have been conducted during and after surgery as per World Health Organization (WHO) guidelines.

The check list according to WHO guidelines is as follows:

Before induction of anaesthesia:
- Patient's identity confirmed
- Patient procedure and site confirmed
- Patient's consent confirmed
- Site marked
- Precautions taken to maintain skin integrity
- Baseline vital signs – pre-anaesthesia
- Anaesthesia safety check completed
- Pulse oximeter on patient and functioning
- Was the patient checked for allergies?
- Does the patient have a difficult airway?
- Is there a record made of estimated blood loss?

Before skin incision:
- Confirm all team members have introduced themselves and their roles
- Surgeon, anaesthetist and nurse verbally confirm patient, site and procedure
- Any anticipated critical events noted and documented
- Where necessary, has antibiotic prophylaxis been given.

Before patient leaves the operating room:
- Nurse to verbally confirm the name of the procedure
- Nurse to verbally confirm that instrument, sponge and needle counts are correct
- Was the specimen labelled?
- Whether there are any equipment problems to be addressed
- Surgeon, anaesthetist and nurse confirm key concerns for recovery and management of the patient.

(Refer to the NCS assessment tool on page 143 – checklist 2.4.3.2.1)

Subjective data

A full family and medical history is taken to know the family better and provide advice based on fact: Information relating to the name the child is called by at home, the family's residence, family circumstances, religion/beliefs/customs that may impact positively or negatively on the child's recovery, the child's friends, if any, the parents' occupation or source of income, relations in the home and the child's schooling if old enough. It is also important to know if the family suffers from familial diseases that could have contributed to the child's illness or could have an impact in future.

The obstetrics/birth history of the child: This includes the antenatal care history that considers whether or not the mother was healthy during pregnancy, if she attended antenatal care in full or partly, if there were health problems in general or in particular related to the pregnancy, and if the pregnancy reached full term. It important to find out if the delivery was normal or assisted, if there were problems experienced by the child and/or the mother post-delivery, if the mother bonded automatically after birth, and if she breastfed. Also find out if the child has been hospitalised before and, if so, why. The information collected will assist the nurse in the management of the mother and child.

Objective data

A full physical assessment of the child is done to confirm or negate the subjective data given.
- The weight and height is to be taken so that medications and anaesthesia dosages can be calculated and also to assess if these comply with the child's expected developmental and growth milestones.
- A full physical examination is done to determine the general health status and to detect any deformities. It is of importance to note the condition of the skin, and hydration of the child.
- Vital signs must be taken and recorded to establish baseline data to be used in the future management of the child.
- Test urine and record results.

Common diagnostic procedures include routine blood tests, for haemoglobin, full blood count and blood chemistry, chest X-rays and an electrocardiogram. More specific diagnostic tests may be carried out, depending on the type of operation and the health status of the patient.

Pre-operative care

The pre-operative period begins at the time the decision to undergo surgery is made, when the child is prepared physically, emotionally, spiritually and psychologically for surgery. It includes admission into the health facility until the patient is handed over to the theatre or operating room nurse. At this stage the child's and parents' fears are addressed to facilitate postoperative recovery.

Where possible, the child should be admitted well in advance to allow for:
- adjustment into the hospital routine
- coping with temporary separation and ensuring that the patient is in a state of optimum physical, emotional, spiritual and psychological well-being prior to surgery
- introduction to the treatment that might seem threatening to the child, such as IV therapy and injections
- objective assessment and diagnostic tests and correction of those aspects that might interfere with post-surgery recovery
- if possible, pre-operative theatre visits, even by the theatre nurse. Where this is not possible, a video of the theatre room might be shown, depicting the people in the theatre and the activity in the theatre room.

In elective surgery, the pre-operative care may extend over a period of time, while in emergency surgery the pre-operative care may be short, as the operation is performed sooner.

Pre-operative risk factors

Surgery involves an inherent risk to the patient, no matter how minor the procedure. Surgical risk increases with the extent and complexity of the procedure. Certain patient factors may further increase the risk, such as age and general health.

Age

Very young children have a significantly increased risk when undergoing surgery. The circulatory and renal systems of infants are immature, making it more difficult for them to cope with the stress of surgery.

General health

A patient in good health is better able to withstand the stress of surgery than one who is in poor health. For example:
- Pre-existing pulmonary conditions increase the risk of postoperative lung complications. Children with oesophageal atresia with or without tracheal fistula are at risk of inhalation pneumonia.
- Cardiac conditions may impair the ability of the body to maintain adequate circulation and blood pressure during surgery. For example, children with transposition of the great blood vessels are at risk of circulatory failure.
- Anaemia may be an indication of poor nutrition and, when present, will compromise wound healing.
- Septic lesions anywhere on the body increase the risk of wound infection postoperatively.
- Deficiency of the immune system lowers the patient's resistance and increases the risk of infection postoperatively, for example, patients who are immunocompromised, who have recently undergone radiation, or who are taking steroids or immunosuppressive drugs are at risk of infection and poor recovery postoperatively.

Nutrition

Poor nutrition may retard wound healing. Undernutrition, in particular, lowers the patient's resistance, increasing the risk of infection.

Hydration

Surgical procedures may induce fluid loss and electrolyte imbalance, so it is critical for the hydration to be optimal.

Anxiety

As stated earlier, children may be fearful of hospitalisation and its associated painful treatments. It is important to reassure the child that parents will be allowed to stay with the child as long as is possible and that pain and discomfort will be kept to a minimum and that all effort will be made to reduce stress and strain.

The extent of the procedure
The risk is always increased if the procedure is long or extensive because of prolonged exposure to anaesthetic and other inhalants.

3.1 Pre-operative visits by the theatre personnel

During the 24 hours immediately prior to the surgery, the anaesthetist examines the patient in order to determine the type of anaesthetic to be given, and also to ascertain whether any special procedures or techniques will be needed intraoperatively. The anaesthetist will prescribe premedication, which will be given about 15 minutes before the patient goes to theatre, or when instructions are phoned through from theatre. The anaesthetist may also prescribe night sedation for the patient to facilitate a good night's rest. The nurse should make the results of all diagnostic and laboratory tests carried out on the patient available, including a record of vital signs with blood pressure, weight, height and urinalysis. The anaesthetist's examination of the patient will include assessing the following aspects:
- The age, sex, and weight of the patient to calculate medication dosages and fluid amounts
- Any inflammation of the throat, as this may indicate respiratory tract infection, or laryngitis, which could make intubation difficult
- The patient's temperature, pulse and respiration, and blood pressure
- Any known allergies or a family history of allergy
- A urinalysis that may reveal glycosuria, ketonuria, proteinuria or haematuria
- Confirming the site to be operated upon.

The surgeon visits the patient to answer any questions from parents and patient if possible and to give reassurance, and to check for any last-minute problems. The theatre nurse should further ensure that:
- The patient's records are complete and the consent for the operation and anaesthesia has been signed
- A care plan for safe and efficient intraoperative care has been developed
- The site to be operated on has been confirmed
- A physiotherapist may visit the patient to make sure that they will be able to work on the small body postoperatively.

Legal and ethical issues in pre-operative care
Informed consent for operation
Informed consent is the agreement between the parent or guardian and surgeon for an operation to be performed on the child following a thorough explanation by the surgeon and a complete understanding of the nature of the surgical procedure, treatment options, benefits and risks involved. This informed consent is required for all invasive procedures, no matter how minor the procedure. It serves to protect the patient's right to self-determination and autonomy regarding surgical intervention. Obtaining consent is the doctor's responsibility. The nurse must confirm that the doctor has discussed the proposed surgery with the parents/guardian.

Informed consent may be given by the clinical/chief executive officer, the medical superintendent or their deputy or the magistrate in an emergency where the parent/guardian is not available to sign the consent or, the patient, who, although available, cannot give the consent because of the status they are in.

In terms of the Children's Act 38 of 2005 a magistrate may give consent in respect of minors where the parents or the child's legal guardian refuse consent, and surgery is in the best interest of the child.

Telephonic consent. Telephonic consent may be obtained from a patient's next of kin or legal guardian in the case of an emergency, where the next of kin or legal guardian can be contacted, but may take some time to reach the hospital. In all instances of telephonic consent, a second person must listen to the consent being given over the telephone, and the next of kin or legal guardian must be requested to come to the hospital, with a view to obtaining written consent as soon as possible.

Legal requirements for a valid consent

It is the nurse's responsibility to ensure the validity of the consent. An operation may only be carried out on a patient if the consent given is legally valid. The important components of the consent form include:
- The patient's full legal names
- The surgeon's name and signature
- Specific procedure/s to be performed
- Signature of the patient, next of kin or legal guardian and date
- Witness/es and date.

The nurse should ensure that the following factors are taken into consideration in order to meet the legal requirements for a surgical consent:
- *Sufficient information to comply with the requirements of the National Health Act 61 of 2003.* Entering the proposed surgical procedure on the consent form is a potential legal liability, and, if carried out by a nurse, must be done with great circumspection. The nurse should take particular care of descriptive words such as left, right, ventral, dorsal, total, partial, hemi, etc. to indicate the site or the limb to be operated upon
- *The legal capacity of the patient or the person acting on behalf of the patient to give consent.* The consent must be properly signed and witnessed by legally competent persons. Of importance is that the signing as a witness means that one has personally witnessed the entire procedure of obtaining consent, and that one is satisfied that

> **Practice alert!**
> Factors to ensure that the correct procedure is followed in giving informed consent:
> - Check that the patient was legally entitled to give informed consent
> - The doctor/nurse doing the procedure has appropriately completed the informed consent form
> - The exact nature of the operation/procedure/treatment is written on the consent form
> - The patient's full names are written on the consent form
> - The consent form is signed by the patient or parent/guardian as appropriate for children
> - The consent form is signed by the healthcare provider performing the procedure
> - The consent form is signed by two witnesses
> - The consent form is dated
> - The information is legible.

the patient is giving informed consent and the consent is valid
- *No coercion of the patients to sign consent.* Where the patient does not sign the consent, the relationship to the patient of the person signing must be stated on the form. In the case of consent being given by the medical superintendent or a magistrate, the capacity of the signatory must be stated on the form
- *Record of telephonic consent.* If the consent is telephonic, the form must show the name of the person giving the consent, as well as their relationship to the patient. The form must show the date and time of obtaining consent, as well as the time allowed for the written validation of the telephonic consent. The doctor and the witness must legibly countersign the consent form. The doctor and the witness must both have listened to the person giving their consent on the other end of the telephone
- *No manipulation of information to obtain consent.* Where the patient does not sign the consent, the relationship to the patient of the person signing must be stated on the form. In case of consent being given by the medical superintendent or a magistrate, the capacity of the signatory must be stated on the form.

> **Clinical alert!**
>
> Consent must be signed pre-operatively, before the administration of any sedation or premedication. It must be dated and must give the exact nature of the procedure to be performed. If relevant, the position of and on the body part, organ or limb to be operated on must be specified.

3.2 Medico-legal hazards relating to consent for surgery

Special medico-legal hazards relating to consent forms that the nurse should be aware of may include:
- the form has not been properly filled in
- the form does not specify the procedure to be performed
- the person signing is not legally competent to sign that consent form
- the form has been signed by a person not legally authorised to act as a guardian of a minor, such as the partner of a parent who is not the biological parent of the child
- the form has been signed after the premedication has been given
- the signature is not properly witnessed, or the surgeon obtaining the consent is not the one who performs the operation
- a single consent is being used for more than one procedure – each surgical procedure must have a separate consent form
- improper procedures in the case of a medical superintendent or magistrate's consent are followed
- only one person has taken the telephonic consent
- the form is not dated, or has been dated after the surgical procedure has been carried out
- the form has been signed under coercion, or the patient does not understand what he or she is signing for. Although it is difficult to prove coercion in a court of law, it should be kept in mind as a possibility.

The day of surgery

Final preparation and care of the patient on the day of the operation takes place about two hours before surgery. The parent/guardian's and in some instances the child's anxiety is at its highest. It is important to:
- explain the preparation and procedures that need to be carried out prior to the operation. Also explain about theatre clothes, transport to theatre and the theatre's holding area, as well as accompanying the child to theatre if possible. This is done in an effort to allay anxiety.
- Give an ordinary bath or antiseptic bath if required by the surgeon, and change the patient's clothes to a clean surgical gown and cap. Keep the child warm at all times. The clothes are removed just prior to the operation.
- Remove all jewellery such as little earrings or wrist bangles that the child might be wearing. Jewellery and other valuables must be locked up safely prior to leaving the ward, or given to the parents/guardians for safe keeping.
- Measure and record the weight, height and blood pressure on the morning of the operation to assist in the calculation of drugs and fluids to be administered during anaesthesia and postoperatively.
- Vital signs are taken and recorded, as well as the results of a urine test done on the morning of the operation.
- The patient must be adequately identified by name, hospital admission registration number, name of surgeon, ward or unit, and the procedure to be done. The name must be verified with the patient, if possible. Allergies and risk factors should also be identified. Allergies should be indicated in red on the bed chart.
- All pre-operative procedures such as catheterisation, passing of a nasogastric tube and skin preparation must be complied with as prescribed and recorded.
- Premedication is given at the specified time, or when the instruction is relayed from theatre, and recorded according to institutional policy. It is common practice for prescribed premedication to be given when the order is phoned through from theatre, or when the theatre trolley arrives, as it will still be some time before the operation commences. This is to accommodate delays that may be encountered with the theatre schedule. After the patient has been given the premedication, they must be left undisturbed, as the premedication may contain a sedative. The nurse should strap the patient onto the theatre trolley, or put up the cot bed sides, to safeguard against the patient falling out of bed while sedated.
- Assemble all records (bed letter, observation and fluid charts, blood results, consent form, pre-operation form, blood requisition form, labelled laboratory forms and specimen bottles (if this is indicated) and X-rays that must accompany the patient to theatre, as well as any blood or blood products that may have been ordered.

Transportation of the patient from the ward to the operating theatre

When the time comes for the patient to go to theatre, the theatre will send a porter with a written slip that has the patient's name, hospital admission registration number, name of surgeon, ward or unit, date, the procedure to be done and a space to indicate the time the patient left the ward. The nurse who releases the patient signs the slip and gives it back to the theatre porter. A ward nurse will accompany the patient, together with the theatre porter, to the theatre; or in other instances, the theatre nurse will come to the ward with the porter to collect the patient. On transfer to the theatre, the accompanying nurse must make sure that the patient is securely strapped to the trolley to prevent falls. When the patient arrives at the theatre, the accompanying nurse should hand over the patient to the theatre staff. The consent form must be shown, and the report of the vital signs and urinalysis, as well as details of all procedures carried out in the immediate pre-operative phase, must be given to the theatre nurse. The patient identification must be shown and verified with the theatre staff and the time and type of premedication given must be reported. All other accompanying documents must be handed over. The slip for the delivery of the patient to the theatre must be signed by the theatre nurse, indicating the time when the patient was received. The ward and theatre nurses should ensure that the pre-operative checklist has been completed. In some instances, the parent/guardian may be allowed to remain with the child in the holding area and/or wait in the waiting room if they wish.

Conclusion

The nurse is responsible for the safety of the patient during the preparation for and delivery of pre-operative care. This includes responsibility for environmental hygiene. Surgical procedures may vary according to extent, objective and character; however, the basic principles of pre-operative care remain the same. Nurses should thus develop competence in the assessment and management of actual or potential risk factors pre-operatively, as this will ensure a successful perioperative experience for the patient. Legal considerations, such as the Scope of Practice (SANC) of the registered nurse, authorises the nurse to participate in the preparation for and assistance with operative and diagnostic procedures. The meeting of the full spectrum of bio-psychosocial needs is relevant in caring for the surgical patient, as authorised by the Scope of Practice.

> **Practice alert!**
>
> Failure to adhere to established guidelines or standards of practice pre-operatively that guide patient care postoperatively is a general problem of negligence in clinical practice that can lead to litigation. This includes failure to do the following:
> - test urine and report abnormal properties
> - check that a valid and legal consent document has been signed
> - check and report previous allergic responses of the patient to some chemicals, medications and even wound dressing materials
> - identify or check identity tags, allergy bands, the physical condition of the patient and the operation site
> - monitor vital signs and other parameters
> - keep concise, accurate and properly signed patient care records.

3.3 Medico-legal hazards in pre-operative preparations

Medico-legal hazards relating to immediate pre-operative preparation may include:
- **Inadequate skin preparation.** The patient's skin may be nicked or excoriated during skin preparation. A nicked or excoriated skin increases the chances of infection.
- **Starving instructions not implemented.** The patient may not have been starved for an adequate length of time, increasing the chances to vomit and inhale the vomitus.
- **Premedication errors.** Failure to give premedication, or giving the wrong premedication or a wrong dosage.
- **Incorrect handling of valuables.** Valuables such as earrings left unattended in the patient's locker at the side of the bed and not locked up safely. This exposes the institution to legal action, because valuables may be stolen or lost.
- **Vital signs.** Failure to report abnormal vital signs, or other physical problems.
- **Pre-operative orders.** Failure to carry out special pre-operative orders or orders carried out inadequately.
- **Patient identification.** Inadequate patient identification or patient not identified at all.
- **Consent.** Invalid consent.
- **Falls.** The patient may fall out of bed, or fall off the theatre trolley while sedated, because cot sides were not closed or available, or the patient was not strapped on the theatre trolley securely.
- **Incorrect records.** The wrong patient, wrong patient's records, wrong blood or X-ray may be sent to theatre or the patient's records may be incomplete.

Suggested activities for learners

Activity 3.1
Sindile, 5 years old, is booked for an appendicectomy. He was admitted the day before the operation with pain in the lower right quadrant. The temperature was moderately high. Explain the pre-operative care for this child to enhance healing postoperatively.

References

Child Care Act 74 of 1983. Pretoria: Government Printers.
Children's Act 38 of 2005. Pretoria: Government Printers.
Constitution of the Republic of South Africa Act 108 of 1996. Pretoria: Government Printers.
Harrison, V. 2012. *The newborn baby*. 6th edition. Cape Town: Juta.
Hockenberry, MJ & Wilson, D. 2015. *Wong's nursing care of infants and children*. 10th edition. Elsevier.
Mogotlane, S, Mokoena, J, Chauke, M, Matlakala, M, Young, A & Randa, B. 2018. *Juta's complete textbook of medical surgical nursing*. 2nd edition. Cape Town: Juta.

Mott, SR, James, SR & Sperhac, AM. 1990. *Nursing care of children and families.* 2nd edition. New York: Addison-Wesley Nursing.

National Health Act 61 of 2003. Pretoria: Government Printers.

Patients' Rights Charter. National Department of Health. http://www.doh.gov.za/docs/legislation/patientsright/chartere.html.

4 Intraoperative nursing care of children

LEARNING OBJECTIVES

On completion of this Chapter, you should be able to:
- describe the intraoperative nursing care of a patient undergoing surgery
- create and maintain a therapeutic and safe environment in the operating room, designed to facilitate surgery and recovery from surgery
- describe the different roles of nurses in theatre
- recognise and manage intraoperative complications.

KEY CONCEPTS AND TERMINOLOGY	
anaesthesia:	A loss of feeling or sensation of pain induced by anaesthetic agents such as drugs or inhaled gases.
anaesthetic nurse:	The nurse who assists the anaesthetist directly with induction of anaesthesia to the patient.
anaesthetist:	The doctor who administers anaesthesia to the patient who is undergoing a surgical procedure.
circulating nurse:	The nurse who counts swabs and is available to replenish items on the operating table.
intraoperative period:	The period from when the patient is transferred to the operating theatre table until the surgery is completed and the patient is taken to the recovery room.
scrub nurse:	The professional/registered nurse who assists the surgeon directly within the sterile field, by passing instruments, sponges and other sterile equipment to the surgeon on the directive of the surgeon. The scrub nurse scrubs and dons a sterile gown, gloves, a mask and a cap during the surgical procedure.
theatre reception area:	The non-sterile area through which the patient arrives in the theatre. This is where the patient is received by the theatre nurse and the report is handed over by the accompanying ward nurse.
theatre recovery room:	The area to where the patient is transferred for a brief period following surgery. In the recovery room, the patient is monitored and assisted to recover from anaesthesia before being transferred back to the ward.

PREREQUISITE KNOWLEDGE
- Anatomy and physiology of all the systems in the body
- Application of universal precautions, microbiology and parasitology
- The principles of scientific record-keeping

MEDICO-LEGAL CONSIDERATIONS

Nurses are obliged to provide for the safety of the patient during the intraoperative period and to keep accurate and complete records of the patient. This includes ensuring that all the supplies and instruments required in the operating room and in the recovery room are available and in working order, and that the environment, including the circulating air, is free of micro-organisms. The nurse must ensure that the instruments and swabs are all accounted for at the end of the operation and that none of these are accidentally left inside the operation site. Leaving a swab or instrument behind in the operation site is termed gross negligence and can cost the patient his life and the surgeon and the theatre nurse their careers.

It is essential to ensure that infection control measures are in place according to the healthcare service policy and emergency blood products and fluids are available in a designated and appropriate area.

ESSENTIAL HEALTH LITERACY

The operation room and theatre environment as a whole can be very intimidating to the patient, accompanying family or significant other. Where possible, the patient and family should have been orientated to the layout of the theatre and the activities that take place inside, either through a video tape or, in small hospitals, an actual walk through the theatre. This can make the patient and the accompanying family members less nervous. Children coming for surgery, if old enough, need to be informed about the holding area, anaesthesia and anaesthesia induction, monitoring techniques, length of procedure, post-anaesthesia care and follow-up care in the ward. Allow the children and their parents/guardians to communicate any concerns or discomforts if possible, so that appropriate responses can be provided.

Introduction

Surgery takes place in the operating theatre or operating room. The aim of intraoperative nursing care is to restore and/or maintain the health and welfare of the patient during the actual surgical intervention. The role of the nurse in the operating theatre is to assist the surgeon and ensure that the operation is a success.

The theatre environment

The theatre environment has a reception area, the operating room and the recovery room. The operating room is a specific room where operations and other diagnostic procedures are performed. A well-planned theatre should allow for minimal movement, promote control and visibility, and adhere to the principle of aseptic traffic flow. For example, 'clean' and 'dirty' areas (defined below) are kept separate, and traffic flow between these areas is strictly regulated. The theatre suite is located away from the hospital's main entrance in an area accessible to the critical care units, emergency surgical units, surgical wards and central sterilising departments. In a multi-storey building, a dedicated patients' lift near the theatre suites is necessary.

Each theatre complex will have three areas, as follows:
1. **A clean area, also known as a restricted area.** This area contains the change rooms for the staff, through which the theatre staff enter and leave the theatre, the patients' waiting area, offices, tea rooms and storage rooms, as well as the recovery room.
2. **An aseptic or sterile area.** This area contains the operating suites/rooms themselves, which are equipped with all the necessary equipment, and have floors and walls made of a durable, washable, anti-static material. The sterile area also contains scrubbing and setting-up areas and the sterile supply rooms.
3. **Dirty area.** This area contains washing machines for theatre linen and instruments, sinks and drying cabinets. The area also contains autoclaves that ideally should open in the sterile supply area. Dirty linen, instruments and medical waste are sorted and cleaned in this area.

The theatre department must always be air-conditioned. Air conditioning refers to mechanical regulation of the volume, airflow, humidity, temperature and purity of air flowing through the area. Temperature control should be maintained at 20 °C to 24 °C for the comfort of the personnel without putting the patient at risk of hypothermia. The humidity is maintained between 50% and 60% (American Society for Healthcare Engineering, 2013) and is controlled to provide a comfortable environment for the personnel. Humidity levels greater that 60% may be conducive to bacterial growth. Air conditioning control is done through filtering of the air through a High Efficiency Particulate Air (HEPA) filter system. These systems filter out virtually all particles from the outside air before it enters the operating room. Airflow is designed so that clean air enters from vents in the ceiling close to the centre of the room and exits close to the floor at the periphery, carrying the airborne particles down and away from the surgical field.

Communication systems between theatres, theatre manager's office, recovery room and tea room must be linked. An emergency bell between the theatre suites and intensive care units must be installed. Telephones and intercoms are most commonly used. Noise levels in theatres and recovery room must be controlled. Lighting must be diffused and evenly distributed through the theatre to allow sufficient lighting for the anaesthetist and all surgical members of the team. The operating light must give an intense, easily adjustable light, minimal heat, be shadowless and fitted with an adjustable control for focus.

The intraoperative care team

The surgical team in theatre consists of the surgeon, one or two assistants (surgeons), an anaesthetist, a nurse to assist the anaesthetist, a scrub nurse and a circulating or 'floor' nurse to run errands (fetch and carry), and there may be a learner who is an observer. Each of these individuals has a specific function in the theatre room. The recovery room is normally staffed by professional nurses, learner nurses and enrolled nurses, sometimes with an anaesthetist. The patient in the recovery room remains the responsibility of the anaesthetist who administered anaesthesia.

Other health professionals involved in theatre are radiographers, radiologists, pathologists, perfusionists and laboratory technicians. A theatre department also needs clerks to assist the theatre nursing service manager to do theatre bookings. Other subcategories of workers include the following:
- patient management executives (PMEs) such as porters and messengers who transport patients to and from theatre, who may help lift patients and also transport specimens from theatre and collect results from the laboratory or X-ray plates
- general assistants or cleaners to clean the floors and assist with end-of-day general cleaning
- packers and technicians in the central sterilising department.

> **Clinical alert!**
> The support team for the theatre is an important factor affecting intraoperative procedures. The diagnostic tests for patients intraoperatively vary according to the type of operation. Therefore, prior arrangement will have been made to have the relevant team available. For example, the radiologist may be needed for orthopaedic procedures, or the perfusionist for cardiac procedures.

The role of the theatre reception nurse
The theatre nurse has to:
- identify the patient by asking for the full name and surname, if the patient is old enough, before the patient is put under anaesthesia; otherwise she has to:
  - verify the identification of the patient against the hand band and preoperative checklists on the patient's records, for the patient's name, surname, hospital registration number, operation and site of operation (where applicable), and patient's religion (if applicable)
  - verify the identification of the patient against the theatre slip used to transport the patient
- keep the patient warmly covered at all times, create and maintain privacy and reassure the patient
- check for the completeness of the medical and nursing records, ie signed consent for operation (see Box 4.1), identification of any allergies is marked in red across the bed letter page (patient's record), premedication given and time administered; check that prostheses if any have been removed; and check for investigation results including X-rays (plates and records)
- note when the patient last took food or fluid by mouth
- check that the correct theatre clothes are provided for the patient, ie a theatre gown (open at the back and no nylon undergarments) and cap to cover the hair
- assess the patient's physical and psychological readiness for surgery as indicated in the patient's bed letter
- check the mobility and the functional status of the patient to use this as the baseline post-anaesthesia
- keep the patient comfortable and safe with cot sides raised
- accompany the patient to the operating room door by walking next to the bed or trolley at the head end to be in sight of the patient's face and to continuously observe the patient

- hand over and report any recorded abnormalities to the theatre nurse
- if the patient is with the family, direct the family to the waiting area as the child is wheeled into the theatre.

4.1 Checking the consent form

- The consent form must state who is giving the consent and for what purpose (in case of a guardian or parents), for which procedure, and by which surgeon
- The patient's name must be written in full
- The doctor who obtained the informed consent is the one who is going to operate on the patient. Two witnesses must have signed the consent – one witness should preferably be a professional nurse
- The procedure must be written clearly, and no abbreviations may be used
- Where applicable, the site to be operated on must be stated clearly
- The patient or guardian's signature should be legible, and the capacity of the person signing the consent form indicated.

The role of the scrub nurse

In the theatre, the role of the scrub nurse is to:
- identify the patient's needs through a preoperative visit
- prepare the operating theatre, surgical supplies, instruments and equipment in the sterile area
- brief the circulating nurse about their duties during the procedure
- assist the surgeon by anticipating and meeting the surgeon's requirements
- ensure that the patient is protected from medico-legal risks, such as a break in sterility during the procedure
- maintain the principles of asepsis
- control swabs, instruments and needles during and after the procedure
- control consumables used intraoperatively to avoid wastage
- complete all documentation accurately
- ensure continuity of patient care by handing over to recovery room staff.

The role of the circulating nurse

During surgery, the circulating nurse is required to do the following:
- manage the activities outside the sterile area
- assist in the preparation of the theatre for surgery
- ensure that the scrub area is clean and properly stocked
- keep the setting room clean and tidy
- open sterile packs and supplies aseptically
- control instruments, swabs and needles with the scrub nurse
- handle specimens correctly
- tidy and clean the operating room between cases
- clean and stock the operating room at the end of the operations
- assist with the care and safety of the patient by preventing medico-legal risks

- prevent the spread of infection by ensuring asepsis and upholding the principles of cross infection
- keep accurate record of all consumables used intraoperatively.

The role of the anaesthetic nurse

In the theatre it is important for the anaesthetic nurse to:
- prepare the anaesthetic requirements to ensure patient safety, including emergency equipment and drugs, defibrillator and emergency trolley
- depending on the age of the patient, explain the procedure to the patient and remain in the theatre with the patient and the anaesthetist
- ensure a safe and comfortable environment for the patient undergoing anaesthesia and during the operation period
- protect the patient from any physical discomfort or embarrassment before, during and after the administration of anaesthesia
- assess the patient for potential complications and abnormal stress responses and report to the anaesthetist and scrub nurse
- connect and check the anaesthetic machine, gases, laryngoscopes, endotracheal tubes, suction equipment, monitoring equipment and ventilator
- control the drugs used during each procedure. Many of the drugs are scheduled substances and must be carefully controlled and accounted for in a scheduled substance register
- assist the anaesthetist with induction, maintenance and completion of anaesthesia.

Reception of the patient in the operating room

Once inside the theatre, the patient should not be left unattended. The patient must again be properly identified when transferred onto the operating table and the operative site must be checked and confirmed. Another identification is by the scrub nurse, who verifies the name against the identity band and the bed letter or folder and hospital number. The consent document is checked again for signatures. The type and site of surgery are confirmed. The anaesthetic nurse checks for allergies, last oral intake and whether premedication was administered to the patient and the time it was administered.

4.2 Steps to be followed upon receiving the patient in the operating room

- Ensure safety during transfer of the patient from the bed to the operating table
- If patient is old enough, confirm the exact nature of the proposed procedure (as recorded on the consent form) with the patient on transfer to the operating table
- Check allergy bands and previous allergic responses of the patient to anaesthesia and other medications, including contrast media
- Check identity tags, physical condition of the patient, and confirm the operation site
- Check that blood has been ordered for the patient preoperatively, in case this is needed intraoperatively.

4.3 Surgical positions and pressure points

Some common surgical positions and their potential pressure points are as follows:
- **Supine (dorsal recumbent) position with the head gently turned to the side.** Occiput, scapula, thoracic vertebrae, olecranon, sacrum and coccyx, and calcaneus.
- **Prone position.** Cheek and ear, acromion process, breasts in females, genitalia in males, patella and toes.
- **Lateral position.** Ear, acromion process, ribs, ileum, greater trochanter, medial and lateral condyles, and malleolus.
- **Lithotomy position.** Peroneal nerve, femoral nerve, obturator nerve and popliteal space.

Positioning the patient on the operating table
The position of the patient must be as natural as is possible to avoid injury and pressure to delicate structures, yet allow for adequate access by the surgeon and the anaesthetist.

Induction of anaesthesia
Induction and reversal of the patient from anaesthesia are the critical points of intraoperative care of the patient. Before induction of anaesthesia, introduce the patient to the anaesthetist. A patent airway should be ensured, and the patient should be provided with adequate ventilation and oxygenation. The safety of the patient should be maintained, because the patient may experience retching, vomiting, shivering, biting of the tongue or restlessness during induction and reversal of anaesthesia.

4.4 Different types of anaesthesia

There are different types of anaesthesia, such as the following:
- **General anaesthesia** is induced for major operations. It is administered through a breathing mask or tube and IV infusion and it causes loss of consciousness, relaxes the muscles and produces amnesia. During general anaesthesia, the patient cannot be aroused and does not respond even to painful stimulus. The patient is not able to breathe independently or maintain a patent airway, and thus is assisted with mechanical ventilation.
- **Local anaesthesia** temporarily stops the sensation of pain at the operation site. The patient remains conscious. It can be administered by injection or application on the site.
- **Regional anaesthesia** numbs only a specific area that is operated upon. Nerve block is achieved by injection of local anaesthesia in the area that the nerve supplies. Bier block is achieved by administering local anaesthesia into the venous system of the exsanguinated extremity. The anaesthetic agent is injected into the veins of the limb while using a tourniquet.
- **Spinal anaesthesia** is where an anaesthetic drug is injected into the fluid in the spinal cord. It is often given in lower abdominal, rectal or lower-extremity surgery.

Recovery room care

The recovery room is an area where patients are transferred to postoperatively and are cared for until the primary effects of anaesthesia have worn off. The anaesthetist authorises the transfer to the recovery room when satisfied with the condition of the operated patient. Patients remain in the recovery room until they have regained consciousness and are able to breathe spontaneously and can maintain a patent airway independently. The objective of recovery room care is to provide safe and effective post-anaesthetic care and to ensure continuity of care. In the recovery room the care of the patient proceeds as follows:

- The identity and condition of the patient is checked; airway patency, breathing, colour of the skin and mucous membranes, responsiveness and level of consciousness are also assessed.
- The patient must be covered adequately and warmly.
- The operation and anaesthetic details as well as postoperative instructions are handed over to the recovery room nurse by the scrub nurse and/or the surgeon.
- The patient is connected to monitoring devices to monitor vital signs.
- Responsiveness is established.
- Oxygen is administered for the first 2 to 4 hours after surgery. The reason for this is that anaesthetic gases are being excreted via the lungs during this period and these gases take up space in the lungs that would normally be oxygenated.
- Intravenous therapy is checked and maintained according to prescription.
- Complications related to anaesthesia or the procedure itself are observed and treated. The nurse should be especially alert for respiratory problems, hypotension, bleeding, as well as nausea and vomiting.
- Pain management in the recovery room is important, because the effects of the anaesthesia may start to wear off and the patient would then require pain medication, even if they appear drowsy and groggy.

Practice alert!

The nurse must treat all patients with dignity and respect at all times, including when they are under anaesthesia. Patients should never be exposed unnecessarily, and should never be spoken about in crude or disrespectful terms. Some patients do not lose their sense of hearing under anaesthesia, especially if a light anaesthetic is used, and are therefore able to recall what was said about them when they wake up.

Before discharge from the recovery room, the following aspects must be stable and satisfactory:
- Level of consciousness: the patient should be arousable even if they remain drowsy
- Blood pressure should be stable and within normal limits for the patient's condition
- Colour and perfusion of the skin should be normal
- The patient should be able to move all limbs
- Pain should be controlled.

The observations and treatment should all be recorded. The anaesthetist should give permission for the patient's return to the ward. It is also important to ensure that the anaesthetist and the surgeon have given written postoperative instructions for pain control, medication, intravenous fluid therapy and dressings before the patient is transferred to the ward. Otherwise the ward staff will have to seek these instructions for the care of the patient postoperatively.

Return to the ward and handover
This is the beginning of the postoperative care. To ensure continuity of care during the postoperative period, there must be an accurate handover of the patient's intraoperative and postoperative details with up-to-date recordings. Discharge criteria from the recovery room must be met regarding the level of consciousness, blood pressure readings, circulation and perfusion as indicated in the colour of the skin and mucous membrane, muscle and pain control.

The following are essential:
- The anaesthetist's signature for the release of the patient must be obtained.
- Intravenous therapy must be kept running according to the surgeon's prescription.
- Tubes such as catheters, drains and drainage bags and bottles must be checked to ensure that these are patent, draining and on correct holders.
- If possible, medication for pain control must be administered before the patient is transported.
- The anaesthetist, the recovery room nurse and the porter must always assist in transporting the patient to the ward.
- The recovery room nurse and the anaesthetist must walk at the patient's head side so as to be able to observe the patient continuously.
- The patient must be handed over to a competent registered nurse or enrolled nurse.
- The type of operation performed, intraoperative details and relevant information, such as sutures, drains, blood and fluid administration, other doctor's orders, patient's condition in the recovery room and medication given, must be read out clearly and acknowledged.
- The X-rays and blood that was ordered must accompany the patient to the ward.

On leaving the patient in the ward, the recovery room nurse must sign the reception book and hand the patient over to the nurse in the ward. The ward nurse must be given a verbal report about the condition of the patient during the operation and in the recovery room, supported by a documented record and must check to verify that all drains and tubes, eg IV fluid therapy, are working before signing to accept the patient.

Intraoperative complications
These can be divided into two stages: during the operation and in the recovery room.

During the operation
Injuries. Falls during transfer of patients from the trolley to the theatre table and vice versa may occur. Thus, care must be exercised when lifting the patient. The assistance of the porters should be enlisted if need be to avoid accidents such as dropping the patient or straining health professionals' backs. Trauma to nerve structures due to wrong positioning and exerting pressure over a nerve may occur.
Burns. Burns can occur from the diathermy machine if not properly set.

Temperature variation. Hypothermia may result from overexposure in the operating room or loss of fluid, especially of blood during the operation, with resultant hypovolaemia and/or hypothermia because of an abnormal response to some anaesthetic agents used.

Fluid imbalance. This occurs due to loss of fluid, including blood, during the operation, or hypervolaemia, where fluid replacement is more than body requirements.

In the recovery room

Ventilatory complications. These may manifest as hypoxaemia, hypoventilation or hyperventilation. All postoperative patients should receive 40% oxygen by mask to reduce the incidence of hypoxaemia. If the patient is slow to regain consciousness, or appears to be hypoventilating, it may mean that the effects of narcotic analgesics have not been fully reversed, and the anaesthetist should be informed. Patients who will require mechanical ventilation for the first 12 to 24 hours postoperatively are usually transferred straight to intensive care, without reversal of the anaesthetic. Non-reversal of the anaesthetic in these patients helps to maintain sedation in the intensive care unit.

Pain. This can be minimised by giving a pre-emptive dose of analgesia during the intraoperative period, by doing a regional or local anaesthetic block of the operative area, or by instituting patient-controlled analgesia, eg morphine or fentanyl. Children of the age group 2 to 13 years are unable to tolerate pain, thus extra effort to reduce pain is required.

Nausea and vomiting. Nausea and vomiting are often more distressing than pain when they occur postoperatively. Antiemetics should be given prophylactically in all patients, especially those who are given narcotic analgesics. The vomiting may lead to pulmonary aspiration. To prevent aspiration, the patient should be placed in the lateral or tonsillar position in the recovery room.

Cardiovascular complications. These could include hypotension or hypertension. Hypovolaemia may be masked by vasoconstriction while in the theatre and may only become apparent in the recovery room. The experience of pain may also increase sympathetic activity in the patient, causing hypo- or hypertension. Bleeding must be stopped.

Shivering. This may be as a result of hypothermia or may be due to the action of inhalational anaesthetics. Although not a complication as such, shivering increases oxygen consumption. Patients must be given supplemental oxygen and be kept warm.

Table 4.1 General nursing care plan of a patient intraoperatively

Problem: Pain	
Nursing diagnosis	• Altered comfort due to pain related to surgery performed, evidenced by restlessness, crying, pallor, and, if old enough and awake, verbal expression of pain by the patient
Expected outcome	• Relieve pain and discomfort

Nursing intervention and rationale	• Assess pain adequately to get baseline data against which to measure progress • Administer analgesics as prescribed to relieve pain • Ensure that catheters and other tubes are secured correctly and are draining, and that IV fluid lines are not blocked, as these may cause pain if not draining or running well, eg bladder distension if the urinary catheter is blocked or pain and swelling if drip is infiltrating • Prevent hypothermia. Cover the patient lightly to ensure correct and comfortable temperature • Help the patient to assume a comfortable position without stretching the incision or pressing on it • Monitor and record vital signs to identify haemorrhage and infection, which could be the cause of pain.
Evaluation	• Pain tolerable • Child lying quietly and is not restless.

Problem: Injury

Nursing diagnosis	• Risk of injury related to falls during transfer to and from the theatre table and while under anaesthesia • Risk of injury to nerve structures due to pressure related to intraoperative positioning • Risk of injury related to burns from the diathermy machine used intraoperatively.
Expected outcome	• Prevent falls, burns or injury to nerve structures. Promote normal micturition
Nursing intervention and rationale	• Ensure enough staff to help transfer the patient to the operating table • Use positioning devices such as side rails, foam pads, sand bags, face guards, air mattresses, etc., to ensure that pressure is not applied to nerve structures during operation and to protect these from being damaged • Positioning of the extremities must not exceed a 90° angle, to prevent stretching and compressing nerve and muscle tissue • If using a diathermy machine, ensure the proper setting and function of the machine and that it is correctly placed on the correct site; assess the skin for integrity on removal of the diathermy.
Evaluation	No injuries related to falls, pressure to nerve structures or burns

Problem: Retention of foreign objects inside the operation site

Nursing diagnosis	• Risk of retained foreign objects in the operated site

Expected outcome	• Render operation site free of swabs or instruments
Nursing intervention and rationale	• Count swabs and instruments that are set on the tray at the beginning of the procedure and as additional items are added, include them in the count; keep a record on the board; count these again at the initial closure after the operation and again at skin closure
Evaluation	• No retained foreign objects in the wound

Problem: Risk of hypothermia or hyperthermia

Nursing diagnosis	• Risk of altered body temperature related to the low temperature levels in the operating theatre, evidenced by hypothermia • Risk of altered body temperature related to a high temperature in response to certain anaesthetic agents as evidenced by hyperthermia.
Expected outcome	• Maintain body temperature within normal ranges by adequate covering
Nursing intervention and rationale	• Hypothermia: Apply warm blankets while in theatre, or thermal coverings during surgery • Keep the patient covered at all times • Control the temperature and humidity of the room • Only expose the area that is operated upon • Infuse warm fluids during operation • Monitor the temperature continuously • Hyperthermia: Remove excess drapes • Administer cool intravenous fluids.
Evaluation	• Patient is warm and body temperature is maintained at 36–37.5 °C on leaving the theatre

Problem: Risk of hypovolaemia

Nursing diagnosis	• Risk of fluid volume deficit related to bleeding during and post operation • Risk of fluid volume deficit related to decreased fluid intake secondary to withholding food and fluids prior to surgery, inadequate fluid replacement during surgery, excessive gastrointestinal losses, and inhalation of dry anaesthetic gases and third-spacing of fluid as evidenced by dehydration, electrolyte imbalance, tachypnoea, hypotension.
Expected outcome	• No undue bleeding from the operated site • Maintain normal fluid balance • Maintain normal blood pressure.

Nursing intervention and rationale	• Administer and record volume expanders as prescribed • Administer and record blood and blood products as prescribed • Administer and record intravenous body fluids and replace electrolytes as prescribed • Monitor and record blood pressure • Monitor and record urine output and that of all fluids, including irrigation and blood loss on dressings • Monitor and record vital signs.
Evaluation	• Hydration is maintained • Vital signs are normal • No undue bleeding during the operation period.

Problem: Risk of hypervolaemia/fluid overload

Nursing diagnosis	• Risk of fluid volume overload related to increased intravenous replacement of fluids and massive blood and blood products transfusion
Expected outcome	• Maintain normal hydration
Nursing intervention and rationale	• Monitor and record vital signs for tachycardia and dyspnoea • Accurately monitor, measure and record intake and output of all fluids • Administer and record diuretics as prescribed • Restrict fluid administration as required • Monitor electrolytes, replace and record as prescribed.
Evaluation	• Vital signs are normal • Normal fluid volume is maintained.

Conclusion

Intraoperative nursing care builds on preoperative care. It requires many technical activities to facilitate the surgical procedure and maintain patient safety, while promoting positive outcomes of the surgery performed. The nurse should ensure and provide a safe environment throughout the patient's stay in the theatre.

Suggested activities for learners

Activity 4.1

You have been allowed to accompany the patient to theatre and to be present throughout the operation.

During the surgical procedure:
• note and record the role of the circulating nurse

- outline the possible medico-legal hazards in the operating room which have to be avoided, and indicate the activities that should be undertaken by nurses to avoid such medico-legal hazards in the operating room
- describe the potential problems that may be experienced by the patient during the intraoperative period.

Submit the case study to the facilitator within a month of completing this chapter.

References

American Society for Healthcare Engineering. 2010. *Briefing for CMS on reduction of low-level humidity in short-term patient care areas.* http://www.ashe.org/advocacy/research/pdfs/briefing_cms_humidity-04-19-2011.pdf. (Accessed 29 November 2018).

American Society for Healthcare Engineering. 2013. *CMS Lowers OR humidity requirement.* http://www.ashe.org/about/ASHE_membership/pdfs/Advocacy_Alert_Sample.pdf. (Accessed 29 November 2018).

Joint Communication to Healthcare Delivery Organizations. 2015. *Relative humidity levels in the operating room.* Joint Commission Online. http://www.jointcommission.org/assets/1/23/jconline_August_14_131.pdf. (Accessed 29 November 2018).

Mogotlane, S, Mokoena, J, Chauke, M, Matlakala, M, Young, A & Randa, B. 2018. *Juta's complete textbook of medical surgical nursing.* 2nd edition. Cape Town: Juta.

5 Postoperative nursing care of children

LEARNING OBJECTIVES

On completion of this Chapter, you should be able to:
- describe the reception and immediate postoperative care of the patient from theatre
- identify the common postoperative actual and potential problems
- design a nursing care plan for a patient based on the postoperative actual and potential problems
- outline the essential health information, including home care for the patient following surgery
- describe recognition and management of postoperative complications
- describe postoperative complications and management thereof.

KEY CONCEPTS AND TERMINOLOGY	
analgesics:	Medications that are given to the patient to treat pain.
aspiration:	Inhalation of gastric contents or blood into the tracheobronchial tree. Postoperatively it is related to decreased level of consciousness, vomiting or inability to maintain a clear airway.
atelactasis:	Collapse of the lung.
gape:	This is when the edges of a wound that had closed during a process of healing separate as a result of infection.
hiccups (singultus):	Abnormal breathing caused by involuntary contraction of the diaphragm and rapid closure of the glottis. It is usually associated with irritation of the diaphragm or phrenic nerve.
hypoxaemia:	A situation where the pulse oximetry is less than 90%, and the partial pressure of oxygen in arterial blood (PaO_2) less than 60 mmHg in the arterial blood.
postoperative period:	This period commences when the patient is transferred from the recovery room in the theatre to the ward or the intensive care unit until discharge.

PREREQUISITE KNOWLEDGE
- Anatomy and physiology of all the systems in the body
- Application of universal precautions; microbiology and parasitology
- The principles of the nursing process and scientific record-keeping

MEDICO-LEGAL CONSIDERATIONS

Every surgical procedure, regardless of extent or objective, involves some degree of risk to the patient. This is true where the patient's potential problems include pain, haemorrhage and restlessness leading to falls, displacing drips, and dismantling suture lines. Postoperatively the patient must be sedated to avoid pain and to keep patient calm. Furthermore, parents/guardians must be allowed to remain next to the child, as they are best able to keep the child calm. The patient must always be nursed in a cot bed with closed side rails, as there may be disorientation following anaesthesia and sedation for pain. The patients' records should be kept safe and always checked for accuracy and completeness.

ETHICAL CONSIDERATIONS

Postoperatively, the nurse has an obligation to:
- note and report anaesthetic and postoperative complications
- monitor vital signs and other parameters postoperatively
- adhere to established guidelines or standards of practice that guide patient care
- keep concise, accurate and properly signed patient care records.

ESSENTIAL HEALTH LITERACY

Small children are often terrified of surgery. They are fearful of cuts on the skin, blood and pain. Therefore, education of both the child and the parents/guardians is necessary in the postoperative period. The child must know:
- how the operated site will look
- that there will be bloody dressings, but the nurse will be there to ensure that they are fine
- the pain will be there, but medication will be given to make it better
- that the injections that will be given will be for the child's good
- that intravenous infusion and transfusion are necessary for speedy recovery.

Discharge teaching of parents/guardians, should cover matters such as wound care, position in bed or when the child is carried around, diet, medications, play, follow-up and the reporting of any problems, as this provides for independence and the ability to take control of events. Personal and environmental cleanliness during the convalescent period at home is important. The parents/guardians must keep appointments for follow-up visits, and must know the complications to look out for. These include persistent pain, restlessness or discomfort of any sort and discharging wounds. Any complications or discomforts experienced must be reported speedily even if this is outside the follow-up dates.

Introduction

The primary purpose of postoperative nursing care is to assist the patient to return to optimum functioning as soon as possible. It involves the care and management of the surgical patient from the time the patient returns to the ward from theatre, until discharged. It may also include post-discharge or home care, depending on the type of operation performed. Some surgical procedures, such as tracheostomy or cleft palate, require long-term follow-up in the community or on an outpatient basis.

Preparation of the environment

The patient must be received into a clean and warm postoperative bed. Many institutions require that the bed be warmed with an electric blanket, especially after major surgery, but the electric blanket is removed just prior to putting the patient into bed. The electric blanket constitutes a medico-legal hazard, in that it may burn the patient. A well-functioning suction apparatus, oxygen together with a suitable oxygen mask, and a complete emergency trolley must be available at the bedside in case of emergency. Observation and fluid balance charts, a kidney dish should the patient vomit, a drip stand and giving set both for transfusion and infusion, Baumanometer and pulse oximeter must be ready at the bedside for postoperative observations.

Postoperative care can be divided into two sections: the immediate care and subsequent care.

Immediate care on arrival in the ward

Immediate care is provided to promote comfort and address potential problems related to the first 12 to 24 hours postoperatively. The nurse receiving the patient must ensure that:
- the patient's records are complete, including all necessary forms which have been completed in theatre by the anaesthetist and the surgeon
- the patient is handed over by the theatre nurse (and the anaesthetist if available) and the report should include:
  - the type of operation done and the findings thereof
  - the condition of the patient during and immediately after the operation
  - any complications during the procedure and how these were managed
  - type of anaesthesia and drugs given during and after the procedure
  - the vital signs on leaving the theatre recovery room
  - the status of all the drainage tubes and intravenous infusion and transfusion lines
  - total blood loss intraoperatively
- there is a written report on postoperative orders, including medications, IV fluids and observations to be done, with the relevant signatures
- all the lines are patent and working, eg the catheter, wound drainage, IV fluid therapy, CVP line, etc.

When this has been done satisfactorily, the theatre nurse can sign off the patient and leave the patient in the ward. Care in the ward includes:
- Establishing the level of consciousness by arousing the patient, calling them by name or looking for responses indicative of consciousness.
- Noting the number and types of lines and drains that are in situ, including intravenous infusion and transfusion lines and ensuring that these are working.
- Checking the wound site for bleeding and drains for amount and type of drainage.
- Noting and recording urinary output.
- Recording of all patient interventions including, where possible, the patient's self-report of symptoms such as nausea and pain.
- Reporting any concerns in writing in the patient's notes and to a senior staff member.

- Positioning the patient on the side if still asleep and condition permits (unless contra-indicated) to prevent the tongue from rolling back and obstructing the airway as well as facilitating drainage of anything in the mouth, such as vomitus or excess saliva. If the patient is awake they may be placed in a comfortable position.
- Taking and recording of the baseline observation data by the receiving nurse. This includes vital signs and blood pressure, colour of the skin and respiratory pattern, the state of the surgical incision or wound, and drainage quarter-hourly. Intravenous therapy should be checked, noting the type of fluid and whether the infusion is running satisfactorily or not.
- The anaesthetist may prescribe oxygen where it is considered necessary and to aid in the excretion of anaesthetic gases from the lungs.
- Checking the postoperative orders and ensuring that these are implemented. These should include postoperative analgesia, antibiotics if required, any other medication, and investigations such as X-rays and bloods as well as intravenous fluids.
- Keeping the patient warm, but not, to avoid sweating, which could be a way of losing fluid insensibly.

Common postoperative problems

Postoperative problems include:
- **Pain and discomfort.** It is very important that the child is not in pain, as this is one aspect that impacts negatively on the child's experiences of hospitalisation:
  - Pain must be assessed every 30 minutes.
  - Sedatives must be given as prescribed and their effectiveness must be gauged against the child's restlessness or calmness.
  - The parent must be in the vicinity when the child regains consciousness. The care staff must make it possible for the parent/guardian to hold the child on their lap and, if the child is able to breastfeed, the mother must be allowed to do so as this will give the child maximum security.
  - Movement must be encouraged and any movement, especially following abdominal operations, must be assisted so as to reduce pain.
  - The physiotherapist must be engaged to assist with therapeutic movement (exercises).
- **Haemorrhage.** The dressings must be observed for haemorrhage. Report any undue bleeding, repack the wound and try and stop the bleeding. Variations in pulse and blood pressure may be indicative of haemorrhage and whenever these are observed must be reported immediately to the surgeon.

> **Clinical alert!**
> Much as children are afraid of blood, dressings and bandages can make them feel important and get the attention of the carers.

- **Fluid deficit and inadequate nutrition.** There is a risk of poor hydration postoperatively based on the 'nil per os' order the night before the operation, the nasogastric drainage to empty the gastric contents and prevent vomiting, postoperatively and sometimes because of blood loss and no food postoperatively for a day or two, depending on the operation done and the site thereof.
  - Children, especially the very young, easily get hypoglycaemic.
  - The nurse must make sure that the intravenous infusions and transfusions are

running as prescribed and the introduction of feeds is to be commenced as soon as the condition permits.
- **Hypothermia.** The nurse must ensure that the child is adequately covered to prevent hypothermia. The hydration must be closely monitored because dehydration might contribute to hypothermia.
  - Monitor temperature, pulse, respiration and blood pressure every 30 minutes in the first 6 hours, hourly in the next 6 hours and, depending on the condition of the child, if vital signs are stable these can be done every 4 hours.
- **Potential for airway obstruction.** This may occur from movement of the tongue into the posterior pharynx when the patient relaxes from anaesthesia. This is managed by putting the child in a lateral position or, in cases of abdominal operations, the child assumes a recumbent position with the head turned to the side.
- **Hypoxaemia from possible hypoventilation.** This may be related to respiratory centre depression, decreased lung and chest wall compliance, abdominal distension and insufficient reversal of neuromuscular blocking agents, aspiration caused by regurgitation, and laryngospasm from airway irritation during intubation or extubation. This is managed by administering oxygen and where there is abdominal distention a nasogastric tube is inserted to facilitate drainage and decompression of the abdomen. In return for better ventilation.
- **Hypotension or hypertension and cardiac dysrhythmias.** These result from the influence of the anaesthetic agents on the cardiovascular system and fluid deficit or overload, respectively. The improvement of ventilation tends to facilitate the excretion of the anaesthetic agents, thus improving the cardiovascular symptoms, while careful monitoring of the intravenous infusion therapy should be mandatory.
- **Elimination.** Encourage the patient to void within 4 hours of returning from theatre, unless catheterised.
  - Monitor urine output by checking nappies for dampness and concentration of urine.
  - Apply warmth over the bladder to relax the urethral sphincter muscle if there is retention.
  - Also increase fluid intake and keep a record thereof.
  - Catheterisation should be the last resort.
  - Monitor bowel sounds and bowel action following general anaesthesia as anaesthetic agents decrease gastrointestinal tract (GIT) motility, making the large intestine sluggish. Reduced food intake and starvation preoperatively also contribute to constipation.
  - Paralytic ileus can also contribute to constipation post gastrointestinal tract surgery or general anaesthesia if feeds are introduced too soon before bowel sounds are heard.

Subsequent care
This is postoperative care following the 12 or 24 hours up to discharge and in some cases extending into community care (see Table 5.1). The 4-hourly observations of the vital signs are continued. This will help to identify problems early, such as:
- **Infection.** Infection of the wound is a potential problem that must be prevented. Other infections could arise from prolonged bed rest, such as prostatic pneumonia.

- Observe the wound for persistent pain, swelling, bleeding and/or seropurulent discharge.
- Monitor vital signs 4-hourly to assist in the detection of infection.
- Attend to the wound according to the doctor's prescription, using aseptic technique.
- Antibiotics may be prescribed, depending on the identified micro-organism growth, where infection of the wound is suspected.
• **Prostatic pneumonia.** This is a problem of immobility. In many instances, immobile postoperative patients do not expand their lungs adequately, an action that can lead to the collapse of the lungs or atelectasis. Atelectasis is easily detected as an opaque area on a chest X-ray, and for this reason a chest X-ray should be done on all postoperative patients following major surgery. Furthermore, secretions are increased due to the effects of anaesthetic agents, but pain and discomfort make the patient reluctant to cough up these secretions. The retained secretions invariably become infected, leading to pneumonia.

> **Clinical alert!**
> Coughing following abdominal and thoracic procedures is particularly painful, as the muscles used for coughing are affected by the operation. Good lung expansion will promote the removal of bronchial secretions and prevent pulmonary complications. A physiotherapist must be engaged to assist especially the young child who cannot voluntarily cough up any sputum.

- Pneumonia and atelectasis can be prevented by effective deep breathing and coughing exercises in the early postoperative phase. In children, the assistance of the physiotherapist is enlisted to help improve respiration and expand the lungs.
- Monitoring of vital signs every 4 hours will help detect respiratory infection early. A raised temperature and increased respiratory rate must be reported to the surgeon.
• **Loss of weight.** This is usually as a result of reduced food intake, pain and reduced activity. Normal feeding should be resumed as soon as is permitted and resumption of normal activities of daily living such as play should be encouraged.
• **Reduced activity.** This is as a result of pain and weak musculature.
    - The child should be kept pain free and encouraged to play. Toys must be put in the cot bed and, if condition permits, the child can be escorted to the playroom and play under supervision so that other children do not hurt the child, or that the child does not hurt itself through careless play.
    - Often the assistance of the physiotherapist is enlisted to move the child carefully without initiating pain. Mobility will assist with respiration as well as strengthen the muscles.
• **Psychological support.** The child as well as the parents needs psychological support.
    - Reassure the patient and provide psychological support, especially to the parents. Provide information on the prognosis following surgery, and answer questions about the progress postoperatively.
    - Maintain interpersonal relations and trust by displaying an attitude of empathy and patience, both verbally and non-verbally. Anxiety may slow down the child's recovery, and therefore reassurance is of utmost importance.
    - Explain progress to the family and involve them in the patient's care. The family is often anxious and in need of support and information.

Late postoperative-period nursing care
Once the immediate postoperative phase is over, the patient will increasingly become more comfortable. The patient will require preparation for discharge. The family will need information on care and must be allowed more independence so that they can themselves judge how much they can do. Their questions must be answered and information must be provided on wound care, feeding, hydration, body hygiene and general observations to identify problems early.
- Once the patient is taking a full ward diet, the nurse should ensure that the patient takes a balanced diet rich in kilojoules, proteins and vitamins, which will aid the physiological processes of wound healing.
- As convalescence progresses, the use of narcotic analgesics, eg morphine, can be reduced and replaced by ordinary comfort measures.
- As convalescence progresses, the nurses' involvement in the care of the child decreases and the parents/guardians become more involved in preparation for discharge from hospital.

Late postoperative complications
- **Infection.** Wound infection in the later postoperative phase is usually acquired through poor aseptic dressing technique, cross-infection from other infected patients or contamination from other areas of the patient's body. Clinical manifestations include pyrexia, pain, swelling and redness around the wound, as well as abscess formation in the area of the wound. The wound might also open up or gape.
    - Besides ensuring aseptic dressing technique, this type of infection is also treated with antibiotics. An abscess may require incision and drainage as well as culture and sensitivity tests for the pus to identify the infecting micro-organisms.
- **Secondary haemorrhage.** Occurs around the 5th to the 7th postoperative day and manifests as bleeding, often significant, from the area of the wound. Secondary haemorrhage is always due to infection and the wound must be considered to be septic. The patient may have to go back to theatre in order for the bleeding to be stopped. Because such a procedure follows more than 24 hours after the initial surgery, a new consent is required.

Complications of wound healing
Rupture of the wound
Rupture or dehiscence of the wound may occur before the sutures are removed, especially where an abscess has formed or following early removal of the sutures. Wound rupture is also invariably a result of infection, although rupture without infection may occur in undernourished patients as well. Breakdown of the wound may involve only the superficial layers of the wound, or may involve all the layers, with exposure of underlying organs and tissues. If the wound is an abdominal one, a complete rupture may result in protrusion of the intestines through the ruptured abdominal wall.
- In the case of rupture of a surgical wound, the wound must be covered with sterile and warm saline dressings. Inform the surgeon. Covering the opening in saline dressings will keep the underlying structures moist and limit fluid loss. If intestines are protruding through the wound, they may be gently replaced if this is possible without using force, and the wound covered in sterile cloths that have been soaked in sterile saline. The

patient must be kept at bed rest and closely observed for the development of shock. The patient will need to return to theatre for emergency treatment, with a new consent form, to have the rupture repaired.

Various complications of wound healing, such as keloid and adhesion formation, may follow surgery at a much later period. Adhesions are most likely if there has been infection of the wound. Keloid formation may result from genetic predisposition and it is also more common following infection and inflammation.

Clinical alert!
Sutures must only be removed when the doctor orders this.

Preparation for discharge and essential health information

Preparation for discharge is a very important aspect of postoperative care. It enables the patient and family to cope once the patient is discharged. The precise nature of the discharge plan depends on the nature of the operation performed and whether any complications have occurred. Specific health education will be necessary at this stage if a permanent change in lifestyle is required, eg care of stumps and how to adjust lifestyle and activities such as schooling, use of a prosthesis on a growing individual and accessing psychosocial support following an amputation. General discharge advice should, however, cover the following aspects:

- **Diet and elimination.** The patient is normally discharged on a full ward diet or normal formula feed or breastfeeding. The nurse must emphasise the importance of established feeding and a balanced diet that is high in kilojoules, proteins and vitamins. The information must take the patient's family situation into consideration. Social workers must be consulted where food security is required.
- **Medications.** These must be taken as prescribed. It is important that the patient completes antibiotic courses commenced while still in hospital. The family needs to know which medications are taken, and when and where possible, the reason why a type of medication is given.
- **Exercise and mobility.** A sensible pattern of rest and activity should be followed, ie the child's play must be supervised and the child must not be exhausted from play.
- **Self-care.** If stitches are still in situ at the time of discharge, the family should be instructed on how to maintain personal hygiene and also on the ongoing care of the wound. If the stitches have not been removed at the time of discharge, the parents/guardians should be instructed on when to return, or go to a clinic, to have the stitches removed.
- **Possible problems.** These are problems that are not necessarily related to the surgery done but may nonetheless be experienced at the time, for example, as a result of separation during hospitalisation. The importance of reporting any problems must be stressed. The child, if old enough to understand, should be advised about common problems and how to overcome them.
- **Follow-up visits.** The parents/guardians should know when follow-up visits to the surgical clinic will take place, and the nurse should emphasise the importance of these visits.
- **Other matters that may need to be dealt with.** These include resumption of usual activities such as schooling, pain management and wound care.

Table 5.1 General nursing care plan for a child postoperatively

Problem: Pain	
Nursing diagnosis	• Altered comfort due to pain related to surgery performed, evidenced by restlessness, crying, pallor, and, if old enough, verbal expression of pain by the patient
Expected outcome	• Relieve pain and discomfort
Nursing intervention and rationale	• Assess pain adequately to get baseline data against which to measure progress • Administer analgesics as prescribed to relieve pain • Ensure that catheters and other tubes are secured correctly and are draining, and that IV fluid lines are not blocked, as these may cause pain if not draining or running well, eg bladder distension if the urinary catheter is blocked or pain and swelling if drip is infiltrating • Prevent hypothermia. Cover the patient lightly to ensure correct and comfortable temperature • Engage the physiotherapist to help support the incision and stimulate coughing to reduce pain and also to prevent stagnation of mucus in the alveoli • Help the patient to assume a comfortable position without stretching the incision or pressing on it • Monitor and record vital signs to identify haemorrhage and infection, which could be the cause of pain.
Evaluation	• Pain is tolerable • The patient is lying quietly and is not restless.
Problem: Distended bladder	
Nursing diagnosis	• Altered comfort due to a distended bladder related to anaesthesia
Expected outcome	• Relieve bladder distention • Promote normal micturition.
Nursing intervention and rationale	• Establish possible cause of urinary retention • Increase fluid intake if permitted • Apply heat on the lower abdomen • Catheterise as prescribed as a last resort • Measure and record intake and output. Where this is critical and the child is not catheterised, the nappy is weighed • Monitor vital signs to assess urinary tract function, especially where catheterisation was done.
Evaluation	• Patient passing urine comfortably

Problem: Risk of infection	
Nursing diagnosis	• Risk of wound infection related to surgery
• Risk of lung infection (aspiration and prostatic pneumonia) related to aspiration following vomiting postoperatively and immobility due to pain postoperatively.
Expected outcome	• Prevent and minimise wound and lung infection.
Nursing intervention and rationale	• Monitor vital signs; take note of and report increased rates and rhythm
• Administer and record analgesics and antibiotics as prescribed
• Maintain asepsis when attending to the wound and report any bleeding, pain and inflammation
• Apply dressing to support the wound
• Monitor and record intravenous infusion to prevent dehydration
• Provide a nutritious diet that is rich in proteins, carbohydrates and vitamins to build resistance against infection and promote tissue repair, or maintain formula feeding or breastfeeding, as these have the necessary nutrients to support tissue growth and therefore wound healing
• If possible and permitted, position the patient in semi-Fowler's position to prevent aspiration if the patient might vomit, as this can pose a risk for aspiration pneumonia
• Get the parent/guardian to hold the child in their lap as soon as is permitted as a way of getting the child out of bed early. This might also serve as a way to calm the child down.
Evaluation	• Patient is comfortable. No infection
• Vital signs are normal.
Problem: Risk of haemorrhage	
Nursing diagnosis	• Risk of fluid volume deficit related to bleeding postoperatively
Expected outcome	• Maintain hydration and no bleeding

Nursing intervention and rationale	- Depending on the complexity of the operation, monitor and record vital signs quarter-hourly in the first 6 hours, then every 30 minutes in the next 6 hours; hourly in the next 6 hours and, if stable, every 4 hours until discharge, so that changes indicating problems can be detected early. For example, a thready pulse might indicate internal haemorrhage or the wound might be bleeding
- Observe the wound site for blood-soaked dressings; if observed, pack the wound and report to the surgeon
- Administer and record volume expanders, blood and blood products as prescribed
- Administer and record analgesics and antibiotics as prescribed, because pain may indicate bleeding while infection may cause disintegration of tissue, resulting in secondary bleeding
- Observe aseptic technique in the management of the wound to prevent infection and ensure that wound drains have drained the wound effectively before removal
- Administer and record intravenous body fluids and replace electrolytes as prescribed to prevent dehydration and electrolyte imbalance, which can compromise wound healing
- Monitor and record urine output and that of all fluids, including irrigation and blood loss, and monitor and record vital signs.
Evaluation	- No bleeding
- Vital signs normal.

Problem: Risk of paralytic ileus

Nursing diagnosis	- Altered comfort due to abdominal distension as a result of the after-effects of surgery and/or general anaesthesia
Expected outcome	- No abdominal distension and pain
Nursing intervention and rationale	- Patients who have had general anaesthesia and/or surgery of the intestines, or abdominal surgery where the intestines had to be handled, should present with continuous nasogastric suctioning to ensure that the gut remains empty, thus reducing peristalsis and ensuring that the gut rests and muscle tone returns
- Similarly, the patient should not be given any food postoperatively until bowel sounds are heard and the patient is passing flatus, at which stage clear fluids in small amounts may be given; the amounts are increased gradually and when these are tolerated, small amounts of soft diet are introduced until a full diet can be tolerated

	• Where there is abdominal discomfort, the abdominal girth must be taken daily to evaluate abdominal distention • Encourage the parents/guardians to get the patient out of bed, and walk about if permitted, to assist the return of muscle tone, otherwise the parent/guardian is encouraged to hold the baby in their lap in a comfortable position, moving the baby while they are supported to encourage exercise • Apply all measures to reduce pain, as pain will prevent the patient from moving freely.
Evaluation	• Patient to report passage of flatus and bowel sounds to be audible before oral feeding can commence
Problem: Risk of anxiety	
Nursing diagnosis	• For the parents/guardians and child, the risk of anxiety is related to knowledge deficit about the surgery and its outcome • For the child, the risk of anxiety can be related to altered self-perception and possible disfigurement following surgery.
Expected outcome	• No anxiety
Nursing intervention and rationale	• Provide parents/guardians with information and explain the pathology of anxiety, causes, manifestations, possible prognosis and possible modalities of care and management to parents/guardians and the child, if old enough to understand • Assess incapacity so that proper referrals can be made, eg for cleft palate refer to speech therapist • Provide parents/guardians with information about available cosmetic surgery, equipment and prostheses that can be used to enhance physical appearance following disfigurement through surgery. Reassure parents and child about prostheses and how these are adjusted to the child's growth and development • Refer to a physiotherapist, occupational therapist, biokineticist, speech and language therapist and other therapists capable of improving function of the affected body part • If possible, encourage the patient and the parents/guardians to talk about their condition and allow them to ask questions and to verbalise fears and concerns freely. If parents/guardians can accept the situation they can assist the child better • Provide counselling for both the parents/guardians and child and refer them to a psychologist for further professional counselling if this is deemed necessary

| Evaluation | • Patient and parents/guardians communicate concerns relating to the surgical condition, its treatment and outcomes freely and accepts the situation as it is. |

Conclusion

Recovery from surgery involves proper postoperative care, emotional support and education of the parents/guardians and the child. Many community clinics have a small theatre suite and theatre staff available to assist in the performance of minor surgery or day-surgery. Whether the surgery is minor or major, done at a day clinic or hospital, to the child and their parents/guardians, the impact is the same. There is fear of the unknown, fear of painful treatments, anxiety about the outcome of surgery and anxiety about post-operative care. In these instances, it becomes critical to impart essential health information to all involved about what to do when and how, so that they are able to cope postoperatively.

Suggested activities for learners

Activity 5.1

Baby Sibusiso Zulu is 4 months old and has had an abdominal laparotomy for hypertrophic pyloric stenosis. On admission, there was a lot of activity because the child had been vomiting and screaming with pain at each and every peristaltic movement. The child was therefore dehydrated and lethargic. The mother (Mrs Zulu) brought the baby to the casualty/accident and emergency department where the child was admitted to the surgical ward. She was very anxious but had to sign consent for the child to be operated upon immediately. She was there when the child was prepared for theatre. She accompanied the child to theatre and waited in threatre for the operation to be completed and walked with the trolley back to the ward. She has not had time to familiarise herself with the ward environment, nor has she had time to meet the ward staff.

Based on the scenario above, outline the baby's post-operative needs and those of Mrs Zulu, the mother.

References

Jansen, A, Nguyen, X, Karpitsky, V, Mettenleiter, M & Loewy, AD. 1995. Central command neurons of the sympathetic nervous system: Basis of the fight-or-flight response. Science Magazine, *27D (5236): 644–646.*

Hockenberry, MJ & Wilson, D. 2015. *Wong's nursing care of infants and children.* 10th edition. Elsevier.

Mogotlane, S, Mokoena, J, Chauke, M, Matlakala, M, Young, A & Randa, B. 2018. *Juta's complete textbook of medical surgical nursing.* 2nd edition. Cape Town: Juta.

Mott, SR, James, SR & Sperhac, AM. 1990. *Nursing care of children and families.* 2nd edition. New York: Addison-Wesley Nursing.

Section 3

Common surgical conditions in children

6 Surgical conditions of the face: cleft lip and cleft palate

LEARNING OBJECTIVES

On completion of this Chapter, you should be able to:
- explain the pathophysiology of congenital surgical conditions of the face in children
- describe the specific perioperative care of each surgical condition discussed.

KEY CONCEPTS AND TERMINOLOGY	
acquired abnormality:	These are abnormalities that children experience during the growing and development process. They are not born with the abnormality.
congenital abnormality:	An abnormality that the child is born with.

PREREQUISITE KNOWLEDGE

- Anatomy and physiology of all the systems in the human body
- Application of universal precautions; microbiology and parasitology
- Record keeping

ETHICAL CONSIDERATIONS

Congenital defects of the face can be very disturbing to parents and, where possible, must be corrected as soon as possible. If these defects are diagnosed before delivery, parents must be prepared for this and must be shown pictures of children with defects of the face. They must also be informed about the possibilities of repair or corrective surgery that can be performed and shown pictures of affected children after repair. The repair is usually done early in childhood.

ESSENTIAL HEALTH LITERACY

Parents are informed that, postoperatively, the child may be restless, cry more than preoperatively and be difficult to comfort. They will be supported by the nursing staff and will be allowed time with the child to calm the child down. They must assist in reducing crying. The feeding might be particularly difficult. Care and patience must be exercised and the recommended feeding method is to be used. Always follow the feed with a drink of water to clean the suture line. Parents are to be informed that the repair of a cleft lip may be done in stages if the cleft lip involves a cleft palate.

Introduction

Surgery in children, regardless of the system, anatomical part and magnitude, is a specialised field of medicine and must be performed by skilled medical personnel. The patient (the child) is small in size and the tissues are delicate. This calls for extra care, as these structures can easily be damaged and the treatment or repair may result in a complex complication. Correction of congenital conditions of the face is planned by a team of specialists to ensure success.

Congenital defects of the face

Congenital defects of the face are the result of malformations during the embryonic development. There are several of these defects, most of which are beyond the scope of this text. Some defects such as choanal atresia (which is a congenital defect where the back of the nasal passage is blocked by abnormal bony structure or membraneous tissue due to failed canalisation of the nasal fossae during foetal development) are very rare. The most common are the cleft lip and cleft palate.

> **Practice alert!**
> A child presenting with an obvious congenital defect must always be carefully examined to exclude other defects that may not be as obvious.

Cleft lip

Cleft lip is a congenital defect of the face (see Figure 6.1). Its causes are multifactorial and affected infants may have a familial history of the defect.

Figure 6.1 Cleft lip

Pathophysiology. The pathology of cleft lip can be described within the embryonic development of the face, where there was failure of fusion of the primary palate during the embryonic stage of development. During embryonic development, facial swellings arise on the frontonasal processes. These processes fuse to form a continuous surface of the external face. The primary palate is formed during the 6th week of embryonic development by the fusion of the medial nasal and maxillary processes. The secondary palate is formed as a result of fusion between the palatal processes growing from the oral surfaces of the maxillary processes.

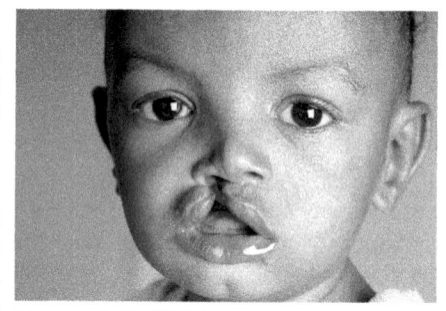

The lip and anterior maxilla develop from the primary palate and complete fusion takes place by the 7th and 8th week of gestation. Each merging or fusion site is a site for potential lip or palatal cleft.

A cleft lip is as a result of failure of the maxillary processes to fuse with the nasal elevations on the frontal prominences to form the primary palate.

- **Types.** The cleft lip can occur alone or with a cleft palate. It can also be a
  - unilateral cleft lip, usually left-sided
  - bilateral cleft lip commonly associated with cleft palate. This is more severe, as it affects both sides of the mouth.

- **Severity.** Cleft lip can vary from a simple notch to a rift that extends into the nasal floor. The immediate impact is on feeding while the later impact is on speech.
- **Incidence.** Cleft lip is common in boys and in children with chromosomal abnormalities.

Clinical manifestations

A cleft lip can be a most distressing feature for a family because it distorts the face of a newborn. The distress can be made worse by the infant's difficulty in feeding, as it chokes and splutters, and if care is not exercised the infant can soon contract aspiration pneumonia. The child may be born small-for-dates and with other abnormalities. These should be excluded on examination. The defect can be repaired.

Nursing assessment and common findings

A full assessment is necessary preoperatively to identify factors that might impact negatively on the outcome of surgery.

Subjective data

A full antenatal and birth history is taken to establish problems, if any were encountered, during pregnancy and delivery.
- It is important to record the health history of the child to establish if the weight gain is as envisaged, and if there are any respiratory infections.
- The extent of the difficulty in feeding must be established and if the parents/guardians have the special long feeding teat or syringe and have mastered the art of using these in order to manage the feeding preoperatively. Nutrition is important, as it will determine the growth and weight gain of the child.
- It is important to find out about the parents'/guardians' schedule, whether they have time to devote to the care of the child. Help the parents/guardians to plan how best to look after the child, because the care will need a lot of time, especially with regards to feeding.
- Parental anxiety must also be determined in the history taking, and coping mechanisms need to be strengthened preoperatively.

Objective data

A child going for repair of a cleft lip will require routine examinations to ensure that they are ready for surgery:
- The child should be weighed.
- Assess baseline data for vital signs.
- Laboratory tests include blood tests to exclude systemic infections and a swab of the cleft to exclude infection on the site.
- Chest X-ray to exclude any chest infection.

Preoperative risk factors for cleft lip

The preoperative risk factors for cleft lip include the following:
- **Age.** The repair can be done at birth, but it is better done at 3 months when the child's weight is stable and there is adequate tissue to breach the gap and parents have learnt how to feed the child.

- **Nutrition and hydration.** The child is likely to be underweight because of the problem with feeding. In many instances, the child cannot create a vacuum for effective suckling, thus feeding requires patience and time. It is imperative that feeding be done using a special teat to ensure retention of feed with minimal waste. This also applies to water given after feeds. This method of feeding will be continued even after the repair operation.
- **Respiratory infection.** This is as a result of aspiration of feeds because of the pathology.

Management of cleft lip

A surgical team assembled for the repair and care of the cleft lip is composed of the plastic surgeon, otolaryngologist, orthodontist, speech-language pathologist, audiologist, paediatric nurse, social worker and psychologist. The team is engaged at different times to ensure success. The repair can be done soon after birth, but it is best done when the child is 3 months old, when it is believed that the child has enough tissue to breach the gap, has gained weight to withstand surgery and the parents have adjusted to the child's defect and are ready to participate in the repair.

Specific preoperative care

The child is usually kept at home with the parents/guardians who are supported by psychologists and social workers. The nurse has to teach the parents/guardians about:
- feeding the child with a special soft, long teat or a syringe to ensure that the child's nutrition is improved and maintained. The use of these feeding methods at home will encourage acceptance of the same postoperatively. If the child's mother is able to breastfeed, encourage her to express milk to keep the flow so that she can continue with breastfeeding postoperatively
- keeping the child in a supine or lateral position with head slightly raised as much as possible. These are the positions the child will assume postoperatively.
- A photo of the child is taken to compare with the repaired version of the cleft.
  For perioperative care, the information in Chapters 3, 4 and 5 applies.

Specific postoperative care

The operated cleft lip is held together with a Logan bow. This is a metal clip that holds the two ends firmly together and it facilitates the union of the sutured edges. Feeding is facilitated with a soft, long teat or a syringe that will not interfere with the suture line. Feeding is followed by a drink of water to wash the milk or formula feed from the suture line to minimise wound infection.

> **Nursing alert!**
> It is important that the child does not interfere with the suture line and the feed does not contaminate the operated site.

Keep the operated site free from blood and serum crusts and gently remove these if present using sterile saline water. It is critical to keep the operated site clean and dry. It is important to try to keep crying to a minimum. Crying will stretch the operated site and might tear the suture line. Paying attention to pain and discomfort is also important, as these elements may cause crying as well. Postoperatively, parents/guardians must spend time holding and talking to the child to ensure comfort and minimise crying.

Restraints may be required by the surgeon to prevent the child from using hands to remove the Logan bow and additional body restraints are necessary for preventing the baby from lying on its abdomen.

Cleft palate

A cleft palate is an oropharyngeal defect that is more common in girls (see Figure 6.2).

Pathophysiology. A cleft palate occurs as a result of the failure of the palatine processes to fuse before the 12th week of gestation, resulting in a cleft of the hard and/or soft palate. The cleft may be unilateral, bilateral or midline. The cleft palate may occur with the cleft lip to produce a complete unilateral or bilateral cleft from the lip through to the soft palate.

Clinical manifestations. These include a visible cleft and difficulties in sucking because the child cannot create a seal around the nipple or teat for effective sucking.

> **Practice alert!**
>
> Use of restraints in the hospital require a doctor's prescription and strict monitoring of the circulation of the restrained arms is vital.

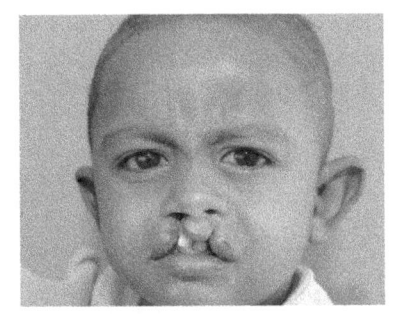

Figure 6.2 Cleft palate

Management of a cleft palate

The management of a cleft palate is surgical, whereby the cleft is repaired in stages. This may commence early, at about 6 months, continuing through to 4 to 5 years, depending on the severity of the defect.

The aim of the management is to:
- maintain a clear airway and prevent aspiration
- allow for the development of normal speech
- provide adequate nutrition.

Specific preoperative care for a cleft palate

Preoperative care begins at home with a focus on feeding the child correctly. The baby cannot grip the nipple or teat tightly and is therefore likely to swallow excessive amounts of air. The feed is also left in the oropharynx and nasal passages. It is important that the parent/guardian is taught and supported on how to feed the baby. The parent/guardian is to hold the baby upright during feeding. A pillow may be used to help maintain this position. A special long nipple or bulb syringe may be used and the baby is burped often to eliminate swallowed air. The baby is given water to drink after each milk or formula feed to rinse the milk from the oropharynx and nasal passages. The baby must be fed frequently and the weight monitored closely.

For the details on perioperative care, see Chapters 3, 4 and 5.

Specific postoperative care for a cleft palate
- Keep the baby in a lateral position to facilitate drainage.
- Suction gently to prevent aspiration from nasal and oral secretions.
- Keep the suture line clean by wiping with sterile saline water to remove any blood and nasal discharge.
- Give small amounts of water every 2 hours to prevent sticky oral secretions while maintaining intravenous therapy for major hydration until the child's oral intake is satisfactory.

Once the child has woken from surgery, feeding is intensified. This consists of clear fluids to be followed by milk formula or solid food as tolerated. Each feed is to be followed by a mouthful of water to cleanse the suture line.

The child's hands are kept in mittens as a form of restraint to prevent the child from interfering with the suture line and disturbing healing.

Figure 6.3 below depicts a repaired cleft lip and palate.

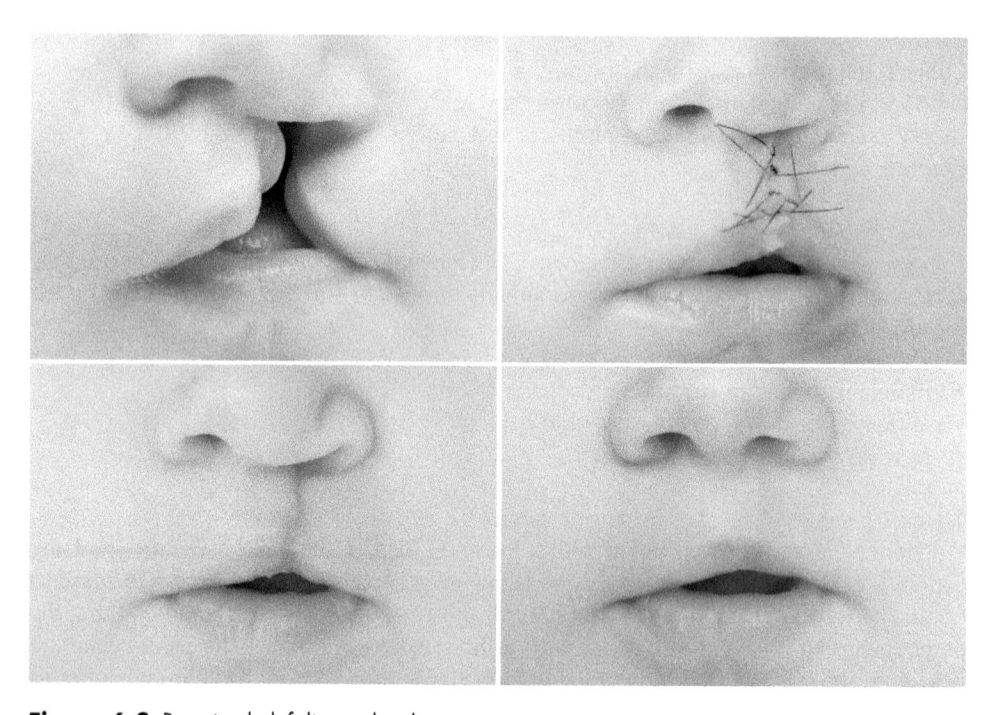

Figure 6.3 Repaired cleft lip and palate

Table 6.1 Specific postoperative nursing care plan of a child who has undergone repair of a cleft lip and a cleft palate

Problem: Pain	
Nursing diagnosis	• Altered comfort related to surgery performed; evidenced by restlessness and crying.

Expected outcome	• No discomfort and pain relieved
Nursing intervention and rationale	• Assess pain adequately to get baseline data against which to measure progress • Administer analgesics as prescribed to relieve pain • Comfort and calm the child by holding, carrying, rocking, talking and reassuring the child that the pain will subside • Allow a parent/guardian to stay with the child to minimise crying • Help the child to assume a comfortable position and keep steri strips or Logan bow in position to hold the edges of the lip ends together to avoid stretching of the incision or pressure on it • Apply elbow restraints so that the child does not disrupt the suture line • Monitor and record vital signs to identify infection that could cause pain.
Evaluation	• Pain is tolerable • Patient is lying quietly and is not restless.

Problem: Impaired skin integrity

Nursing diagnosis	• Risk of impaired skin integrity due to repair done early, mechanical disturbance of suture line, infection of the suture line
Expected outcome	• Suture line is intact and healing well
Nursing intervention and rationale	• Represent the child to the plastic surgeon so that the repair is done at the correct age (at least 3 months or older) • When the surgery is carried out, maintain and supervise elbow restraints to ensure that the child does not pull on the steri strips or Logan bow or the stitches, as this will disrupt the suture line • Position the child in a recumbent or lateral positions to prevent the child from rubbing the suture lining on the bed linen • Keep the child calm and comfortable by allowing the parents/guardians, especially the mother, to stay with the child, hold the child in her lap and comfort the child to avoid crying, as crying might cause tension on the suture line. • Clean the suture line, lip and nostril after each feed as prescribed to remove milk curds and crusting that might predispose the area to infection • A special long nipple or bulb syringe with rubber tubing is used to feed the child to avoid any trauma to the operated site • Monitor vital signs 4-hourly to identify infection early and ensure early treatment thereof.
Evaluation	• The suture line should be clean, free from crusting, intact and healing well

Problem: Airway patency	
Nursing diagnosis	• Risk of ineffective airway clearance owing to oedema following surgery, increased thick secretions, regurgitation due to swallowed air during feeding • Risk of lung infection (aspiration and prostatic pneumonia) related to aspiration following regurgitation of feeds owing to swallowed air during feeding.
Expected outcome	• Child breathing normally, no lung infection
Nursing intervention and rationale	• Change the child's position every 2 hours from back to side and from side to side to promote lung expansion • Elevate the head side of the bed to reduce chances of aspiration should the child vomit • Encourage the parents/guardians to hold the child on their lap to maintain the head-up position and to avoid aspiration should the child regurgitate a feed • Allow child to break wind after each feed to reduce accumulation of swallowed air and thus avoid regurgitation and aspiration of feed that predisposes the child to pneumonia • Monitor vital signs and take note of and report increased rates and rhythm so that lung infection can be treated early and promptly • Monitor and record intravenous infusion to prevent dehydration.
Evaluation	• Patient is comfortable and breathing normally, with no lung infection • Vital signs are normal.
Problem: Inadequate nutrition and hydration	
Nursing diagnosis	• Risk of fluid volume deficit and altered nutrition; intake is less than body requirements owing to the child's inability to suck or take in fluids well as a result of the lip defect and related surgery
Expected outcome	• Hydration and weight appropriately maintained for the child's age
Nursing intervention and rationale	• Provide a nutritious diet that is rich in proteins, carbohydrates and vitamins to build resistance against infection and promote tissue repair, or maintain breast feeding or formula feeding, as breast milk and formula have the necessary nutrients to support tissue growth and therefore wound healing. Ensure non-traumatic feeding by means of a long nipple to ensure that the child is able to suck and retain the feed • It may be necessary to administer and record intravenous fluids and replace electrolytes as prescribed in the first 12 hours postoperatively to prevent dehydration and electrolyte imbalance while fluid and food intake has not been stabilised

	• Monitor the child's weight daily to assess progress made with feeding in terms of developmental milestones • Monitor and record urine output to balance fluid intake.
Evaluation	• Adequate fluid and food intake as indicated by weight gain

Problem: Risk of anxiety

Nursing diagnosis	• Risk of anxiety for parents/guardians and child is related to a knowledge deficit about the surgery and its outcomes • For the child, risk of anxiety is related to altered self-perception and possible disfigurement following surgery.
Expected outcome	• No anxiety for child and parents/guardians. Parents/guardians confirm that they have received adequate information to look after the child at home postoperatively
Nursing intervention and rationale	• Provide parents/guardians with all relevant information and explain the nature of cleft lip and cleft palate, causes, manifestations, possible prognosis and possible modalities of care and management so that parents/guardians are able to participate in the care of the child • Explain the surgical intervention process and how parents/guardians may contribute to the child's care, such as by being available and assisting to calm the child down, helping with reinforcing restraints and maintaining a therapeutic position, assisting with feeding and learning how to look after the child at home • Assess incapacity so that proper referrals can be made, eg for a cleft palate, refer child to a speech therapist • Provide parents/guardian with information about available cosmetic surgery and equipment that may be used to enhance physical appearance following disfigurement through surgery • Encourage parents to talk about the child's condition and surgery and allow them to ask questions and to verbalise any fears and concerns freely. If parents can accept the situation they can assist the child better • Provide counselling for parents/guardians and the child and refer them to a psychologist for further professional counselling if necessary • Keep a photo audit of the child from before repair and throughout the intervention so that parents/guardians are able to visually review progress.
Evaluation	• Parents/guardians communicate concerns relating to the surgery and its outcomes freely and accept the situation

Conclusion

Cleft lip and cleft palate, although distressing to the family, are usually successfully repaired. The child has a prolonged recovery period, with the speech therapist assisting the child to develop speech. The parents also need support for them to cooperate with the therapist for positive outcomes.

Suggested activities for learners

Activity 6.1

Create a nursing care plan for 1-year-old Ntombi, who has had a cleft lip repaired. Use the headings:
- Actual problems
- Potential problems
- Nursing diagnosis
- Expected outcome/s
- Nursing interventions and rationale
- Evaluation.

References

Harrison, V. 2012. *The newborn baby*. 6th edition. Cape Town: Juta.

Hockenberry, MJ & Wilson, D. 2015. *Wong's nursing care of infants and children*. 10th edition. Elsevier.

Mogotlane, S, Mokoena, J, Chauke, M, Matlakala, M, Young, A & Randa, B. 2018. *Juta's complete textbook of medical surgical nursing*. 2nd edition. Cape Town: Juta.

Mott, SR, James, SR & Sperhac, AM. 1990. *Nursing care of children and families*. 2nd edition. New York: Addison-Wesley Nursing.

Skandalakis, JE & Gray, SW. 1994. *Embryology for surgeons: The embryological basis for the treatment of congenital anomalies*. 2nd edition. Baltimore.

7 Congenital defects of the gastrointestinal tract system

LEARNING OBJECTIVES

At the end of this Chapter, you should be able to:
- describe the pathology of congenital defects in the gastrointestinal tract
- explain the nursing assessment and findings thereof
- describe the perioperative nursing care when the defects are/have been corrected.

KEY CONCEPTS AND TERMINOLOGY

anastomosis:	Surgical joining of two parts of a tubular structure.
aspiration:	Inhalation of fluids into the lungs. This results in violent coughing and may lead to aspiration pneumonia.
atelectasis:	Collapse of the lungs.
atresia:	Failure of a tubular structure that would normally remain open to canalise.
fistula:	An abnormal tubal connection from one surface to another that might be due to an incomplete separation or closure of a structure during embryonic development.
ischaemia:	Inadequate supply of blood to a body part
omphalocele:	A congenital defect where the abdominal wall fails to unite in the umbilical area and abdominal contents remain outside in a sac through the umbilicus.
volvulus:	This is when the intestines have twisted on themselves, causing an obstruction and restricted blood supply to the affected area.
pneumothorax:	The presence of air in the pleural cavity.

PREREQUISITE KNOWLEDGE

- Anatomy and physiology of the gastrointestinal system of the human body
- Application of universal precautions; microbiology and parasitology
- Record keeping

MEDICO-LEGAL CONSIDERATIONS

Surgery of the gastrointestinal tract is major surgery and it carries the risk of serious postoperative complications. In children, this is made worse by the immaturity of tissues and function, whereby minimum exposure can result in hypothermia, and a deficit in feeding and/or fluid intake. This can result in fluid and electrolyte imbalance, while early repairs may fail or result in contractures requiring re-operation at a later stage. The immune system is immature, making the child prone to infection. The surgeon has to act with care to avoid medico-legal hazards when operating on children. Where possible, the operation should be postponed to the correct age, when the child can withstand the strain of the operation better. The correct temperature must always be maintained in the environment to avoid hyper- or hypothermia. Where the child has to be starved, a 5% dextrose intravenous infusion must be run at a calculated rate to avoid fluid overload.

ETHICAL CONSIDERATIONS

Conditions of the gastrointestinal tract in children can be congenital or acquired. The surgery to manage the conditions may be an emergency or elective. In many instances the child is usually not able to make any decisions relating to management or treatment. In an emergency, the rush is often risk-laden. The consent form may need to be signed without due consideration of outcomes of the operation, because there will have been no time to give full information. However, rush or panic can lead to wrong actions that may result in negative outcomes. Where congenital conditions can be diagnosed prenatally, it is ethical to inform the parents to expect a problem at birth and discuss planned management with them, so that issues of consent are resolved more quickly when the need arises.

ESSENTIAL HEALTH LITERACY

In child care parents/guardians must always be involved. It is important to put parents/guardians at ease, and this is done by giving parents/guardians adequate information about the condition, the proposed management, the attending doctor, nurse and any other healthcare worker concerned and the part they are to play, and to provide them with whatever skill they will need to play their part.

Introduction

The embryonic development of the gastrointestinal tract begins as an internal tube-like structure, the embryonic gut, which extends from the mouth to the anus. The digestive organs are formed from portions of the embryonic gut, ie the foregut, midgut and hindgut.

The foregut is the portion of the embryonic gut that extends from the pharynx down to the oesophagus, stomach, the duodenum, liver, gallbladder and the biliary tree. The oropharyngeal membrane that separates the foregut from the oral structures disappears, providing for an external opening into the mouth. Failure of these structures to differentiate during gestation may result in defects such as a fistula, stenosis or atresia of any part of the upper gastrointestinal tract, eg in the oesophagus there may be atresia, fistulaa and stenosis.

The midgut is the embryonic gastrointestinal tract that forms the small intestine, the appendix, the caecum, the ascending colon and the initial transverse colon. Failure to differentiate or rotate correctly can lead to intestinal atresias, volvulus or omphalocele.

The hindgut is that portion of the embryonic gut that forms the proximal two thirds of the transverse colon, the descending colon, sigmoid colon, the rectum and the anal canal. The cloacal membrane at the end of the hindgut separates the urogenital structures from the rectoanal structures. Failure of these segments to differentiate and develop may cause colonic atresias or anorectal malformations. Failure in the embryonic innervation may cause aganglionic megacolon.

Congenital defects of the oesophagus and the trachea

Oesophageal atresia and tracheo-oesophageal fistula

Oesophageal atresia and tracheo-oesophageal fistula are congenital developmental defects that may exist as separate entities or in combination. They both involve the failure of the oesophagus to develop as a continuous passage of the gastrointestinal tract. The oesophagus may end in a blind pouch, causing an obstruction (oesophageal atresia) or failure of the oesophagus and the trachea to separate into distinct passages with either forming a linking fistula (tracheo-oesophageal fistula).

Pathophysiology. The oesophagus develops from the foregut, which normally separates longitudinally in the 4th or 5th week of gestation into two parallel passages – the oesophagus and trachea. The passages are joined at the larynx. Defects are as a result of a defective fusion, separation or elongation of the structures.

> **Practice alert!**
> A child presenting with one congenital defect must always be carefully examined to exclude other defects that may not be as obvious.

Types of oesophageal and tracheo-oesophageal defects

There are five known permutations of these defects. All of them pose a threat to life and are considered emergencies. Some of these are not compatible with life. Illustrations of the defects are presented on the next page (see Figure 7.1). Descriptions are included in Table 7.1.

Risk factors include antenatal factors like polyhydramnios, small-for-dates and prematurity. Other developmental defects may also be present.

Clinical manifestations of oesophageal defects

In all the types of oesophageal defects, the affected infant will present with:
- frothy saliva, drooling, choking and coughing. If fed, the child may swallow and suddenly cough and gag, depending on the type of defect
- varying severity of respiratory distress, depending on the type of defect. With type C, D and E there may be distention of the stomach from the air that

> **Clinical alert!**
> Exclude congenital oesophageal defects in a newborn who becomes cyanosed soon after birth, who is drooling, coughing with apnoeic attacks, and has a low APGAR score. Treat this as an emergency. The neonate must be prepared for X-ray immediately and then for surgery if this is indicated by the X-ray.

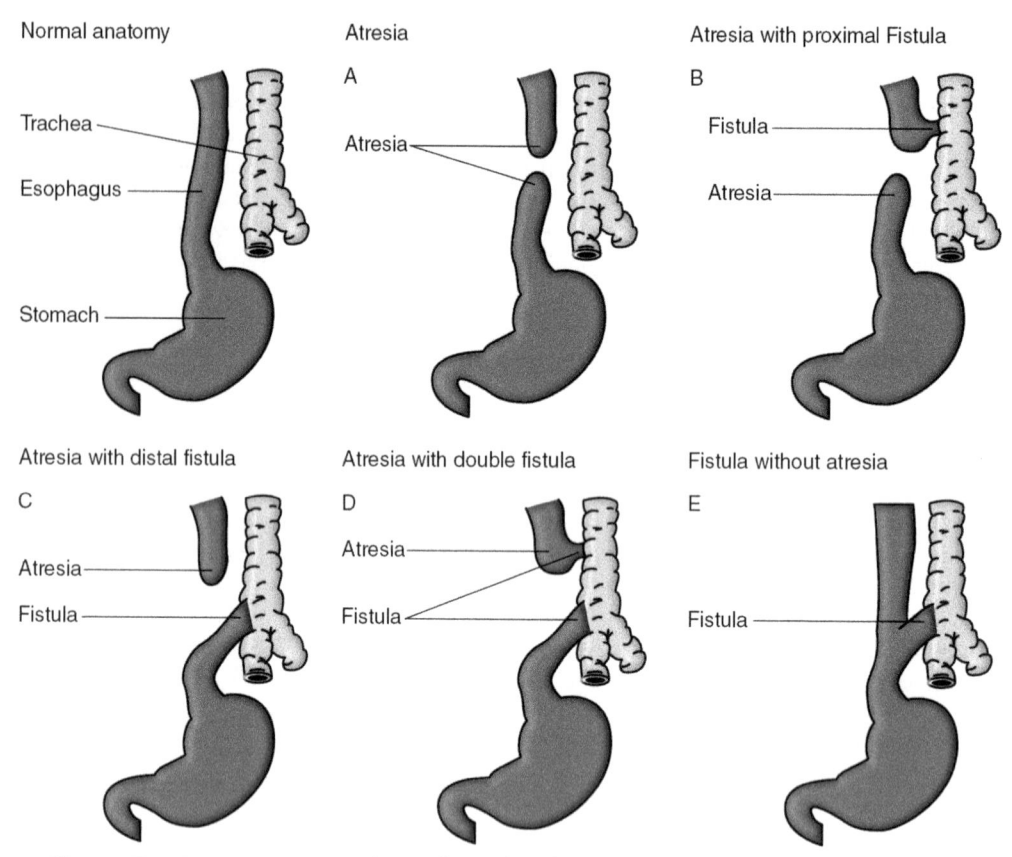

Figure 7.1 Five permutations of oesophageal and tracheo-oesophageal defects

comes through from the trachea and chemical pneumonia from regurgitated stomach contents. For type E (H-type link) cyanosis and choking during feeding may be the only signs, with progressive abdominal distention from air from the trachea.

Preoperative care of a child with oesophageal atresia with or without tracheal fistula
- Keep the infant warm.
- Provide suction through the mouth and make certain that all secretions that can be aspirated are removed and the pouch, if any, is kept empty.
- Maintain intravenous infusion.
- Place infant in an upright position if there is a chance for a nasogastric tube to be inserted, or the head should be lower if it will help reduce the risk of aspiration.
- Provide information to the parents/guardians about the condition and what will be done to correct the defect, the risks the operation carries, as well as successes.
- Obtain informed consent from parents/guardians.

The surgeon may send the infant for radiological examination to confirm the type of defect and to plan for surgery and also to exclude inhalation or aspiration pneumonia.

Table 7.1 Classification of oesophageal atresia and trachea-oesophageal defects

Defect	Description	Characteristics
A: Oesophageal atresia without fistula	The continued development of the proximal segment of the oesophagus was interrupted and it stopped with a blind pouch midway. This is usually at the level of the bifurcation of the trachea. The distal end of the oesophagus has continued to grow down to the stomach. The trachea is normal. The danger is aspiration from the overflow of the proximal pouch into the trachea.	The mother presents with polyhydramnios. This is due to the foetus being unable to swallow amniotic fluid in utero. The infant is either premature or small-for-dates. At birth the infant is drooling and choking on its saliva, and is cyanosed. Immediate management includes: • inserting a short nasogastric tube and leaving it open at the end • suctioning at intervals of 10–15 minutes to avoid aspiration • positioning: upright if the nasogastric tube is in situ; otherwise the head is lower than the rest of the body to allow for free drainage of the fluid that could collect in the oesophageal stump.
B: Tracheo-oesophageal fistula of the proximal segment of the oesophagus and a distal stump that continues to the stomach	The continued development of the proximal segment of the oesophagus is interrupted and linked to the trachea with a fistula, while the distal segment continues to the stomach. The distal portion is continuous with the stomach but separated from the proximal segment. There is a danger of aspiration from anything swallowed, as it flows directly into the trachea.	The mother presents with polyhydramnios. The infant is either premature or small-for-dates. At birth the infant is drooling and suffocating on its saliva, and is cyanosed. The APGAR score is low. This is an emergency. Immediate management includes: • positioning the child with the head lower than the rest of the body to allow for free drainage • suctioning the mouth at intervals of 10–15 minutes to keep the mouth dry of saliva and to avoid aspiration • sending the child for X-rays to confirm diagnosis as an emergency • the doctor may insert a gastrostomy tube to suction out gastric contents and for feeding later.

Defect	Description	Characteristics
C: Oesophageal atresia with a fistula of the distal segment	The continued development of the proximal segment of the oesophagus was interrupted and it stopped with a blind end midway. The distal oesophageal segment is joined to the trachea. The danger is aspiration from the overflow of anything swallowed, including saliva into the trachea from the proximal blind segment of the oesophagus and chemical aspiration from the distal part that is joined to the trachea, as the stomach contents are regurgitated into the trachea.	The mother presents with polyhydramnios. The infant is either premature or small-for-dates. At birth the infant is drooling and suffocating on its saliva, and it is cyanosed. The APGAR score is low. Immediate management includes: • positioning the child with the head elevated, as this will prevent regurgitation of stomach contents into the trachea and will allow for collection of saliva in the blind oesophageal pouch, which can be suctioned out frequently • putting a short nasogastric tube and suction the contents of the pouch frequently to prevent an overflow into the trachea • sending the child for X-rays to confirm the diagnosis and rush the child to theatre as an emergency.
D: Tracheo-oesophageal fistulae without atresia	Both the proximal segment and the distal segment of the oesophagus open into the trachea. The danger of aspiration and that of regurgitation into the trachea is unavoidable.	The mother presents with polyhydramnios. The infant is either premature or small-for-dates. At birth the infant is drooling and suffocating on its saliva, and is cyanosed. The APGAR score is low. This is usually incompatible with life and is an extreme emergency. Immediate management includes: • surgery • setting up an intravenous infusion • holding the baby upright and sending for surgery • insertion of a gastrostomy tube by a doctor to suction out gastric contents • suctioning the child's mouth all the time in an effort to keep it dry of saliva.

Defect	Description	Characteristics
E: Tracheo-oesophageal fistula without atresia	In this defect, the oesophagus and the trachea form an H-type link. This type can go unnoticed depending on the size of the link.	The mother presents with polyhydramnios. The infant is either premature or small-for-dates. At birth the infant is drooling saliva, with episodic coughing and choking, and may be cyanosed. The APGAR score is low.

The surgery performed will depend on the defect, the presence or absence of aspiration pneumonia, and the availability of oesophageal material to do an anastomosis. If there is atresia of the proximal oesophagus, this will be canalised and anastomosed to the distal end to form a passage from the larynx to the stomach. If there is a fistula that links the oesophagus and the trachea, the oesophagus piece that is joining the trachea is ligated to separate it from the trachea and the trachea is carefully repaired to ensure adequate uninterrupted passage of air into the lungs and separation of the two passages. The ligated oesophageal stump is opened and anastomosed to the other distal stump and canalised to allow for free access to the stomach. There may be a need to do a gastrostomy, if there is inadequate oesophageal material to complete the anastomosis. The gastrostomy will be used for feeding while waiting for the child to grow or the anastomosis to heal.

Postoperative care of a child who has undergone repair of oesophageal defects with or without a tracheal fistula
Repair of oesophageal defects is a major operation. It is usually an emergency with minimal preparation of the patient and the family.

Postoperatively from theatre:
- the child will be transported in an incubator for temperature regulation to the high-care ward, where they will remain until out of danger
- there will be intravenous infusion therapy, which must be kept running to maintain hydration and electrolyte balance
- there will be a nasogastric tube inserted to drain the gastric contents and to also minimise the chances of abdominal distension from swallowed air
- there might be a chest tube, if there was any involvement of the chest in the surgery to allow for maximum expansion of the lung
- there might be a gastrostomy tube, which will be used for feeding until the oesophageal anastomosis is healed.

Potential postoperative problems
These include respiratory failure due to laryngeal oedema, atelectasis, pneumothorax and aspiration pneumonia acquired preoperatively.

Nursing management
- It is important that the child is kept warm. Ideally the child is nursed in an incubator.

- Once the patient is conscious, the head is to be put a little higher than the rest of the body.
- When carried in arms, the child must be kept upright.
- The intravenous infusion must be kept running at a prescribed rate to ensure fluid and electrolyte balance.
- The nasogastric tube is to be kept draining according to post-operation orders if there is no gastrostomy tube. The nasogastric tube is kept in until there is no drainage and bowel sounds can be heard. Where there is no gastrostomy tube, the nasogastric tube may also serve as a feeding tube when it is safe to do so.
- There might be an underwater-seal drainage system to assist in the expansion of the lung/s. This needs to be observed for proper functioning.
- Observation of temperature, pulse and respiration is to be done quarter-hourly for the first 12 hours and then half-hourly for another 6 hours, then hourly and 4-hourly as the child settles down. Infection is suspected if the temperature increases and, in some instances in neonates, if there is septicaemia the temperature might be low. Presence of infection is confirmed if there is a purulent discharge from the chest tube or an increased white blood cell count when the blood specimen is checked. The sources of infection could be from a leaking anastomosis or aspiration pneumonia.
- Ensure that the child is pain free by giving the prescribed analgesic and helping the child assume a comfortable position.
- Ensure comfort and calmness by allowing the parents/guardians to stay with the child.
- A pacifier is recommended for a child who is going to be on parenteral feeding for a prolonged period of time to ensure that the child receives oral stimulation.

Table 7.2 Specific postoperative nursing care plan for a child who has undergone repair of congenital oesophageal atresia with or without tracheal fistula

Problem: Respiratory failure	
Nursing diagnosis	• Altered breathing related to ineffective airway clearance, potential for aspiration, impaired gas exchange and distended abdomen evidenced by restlessness, poor skin color (cyanosis and pallor)
Expected outcome	• Breathing rate, rhythm and depth normal for child's age
Nursing intervention and rationale	• Put the child in a comfortable position that will allow for maximum chest expansion. This may be a high-Fowler's position to prevent regurgitation of abdominal contents • A nasogastric tube is to be kept draining into a bag until there is no drainage and bowel sounds can be heard to prevent undue abdominal distension • Ensure that the underwater seal drainage is draining and functioning well to assist with expansion of the lungs. • Monitor respiration and record the rate in graph form to assess progress in improvement of respiration as well as to detect and treat infection early if suspected • Monitor oxygen as prescribed

	• Administer analgesics as prescribed to ensure that the child is free of pain and relaxed • Record any cyanotic attacks, as these dictate the degree of respiratory distress experienced • Engage a physiotherapist for passive exercises to help with lung expansion and improved air intake.
Evaluation	• Respiratory rate is within normal range, indicating improved expansion of the lungs. No cyanotic attacks. Vital signs are normal

Problem: Risk of infection

Nursing diagnosis	• Risk of wound infection related to surgery • Risk of lung infection (prostatic and aspiration pneumonia) related to atelectasis.
Expected outcome	• Prevent and minimise wound and lung infection
Nursing intervention and rationale	• Monitor vital signs and take note of and report increased breathing rate and rhythm • Administer and record analgesics and antibiotics as prescribed • Maintain asepsis when attending to the wound and report any bleeding, pain and inflammation • Apply dressing to support the wound • Monitor and record intravenous infusion to prevent dehydration • Provide breast milk or formula feed in a bottle with a big hole to reduce the sucking effort. The breast milk or formula has the necessary nutrients to support tissue growth therefore wound healing.
Evaluation	• Get parents/guardians hold the child on their lap as soon as is permitted as a way of getting the child out of bed early. This might also serve as exercise to improve circulation as well as a way to calm the child down

Problem: Hydration and nutrition

Nursing diagnosis	• Risk of fluid volume deficit, altered electrolyte balance and altered nutrition related to preoperative care, which requires that the child takes nothing orally, nasogastric suctioning pre- and postoperatively, and poor feeding postoperatively
Expected outcome	• Maintain normal hydration and normal nutrition
Nursing intervention and rationale	• Administer and monitor intravenous fluids as prescribed to maintain hydration and electrolyte balance. Record fluid intake • Ensure that the nasogastric tube is draining and record the drainage as fluid output. Leave the nasogastric tube in situ until there is no drainage, bowel sounds are heard and the child is stable

	• When bowel sounds are heard, gastrostomy feeds are commenced with clear fluids. When these are tolerated, formula feeds are gradually introduced to avoid distension of the stomach
• The open end of the gastrostomy tube is elevated to above the child's stomach to avoid backflow, but left open to allow air to escape
• Gastrostomy feeds are continued until the oesophageal anastomosis is healed
• Oral feeds are commenced when the anastomosis is considered healed. Start with small sips of clear fluids, followed by expressed breast milk or formula to allow the child to learn to swallow
• There may be continued drooling, so keep the child dry by wiping gently and in some instances applying protective ointment for skin care
• Weigh the child daily to assess progress in growth and development
• Measure the abdominal girth daily to detect abdominal distension.
Evaluation	• Child is well-hydrated and gaining weight as expected

Problem: Hypothermia

Nursing diagnosis	• Risk of altered thermoregulation related to the surgery
Expected outcome	• Body temperature is maintained at 36.5–37.5 °C
Nursing intervention and rationale	• Nurse the child in an incubator at a regulated temperature that is monitored hourly to keep the child's temperature at 36.5–37.5 °C. The incubator can also provide for phototherapy if there are signs of physiologic jaundice
• Monitor the child's vital signs 4-hourly to prevent hypothermia that may compromise the child's immunity
• Feed child regularly to provide energy and promote tissue repair.
Evaluation	• Child's temperature is normal

Problem: Risk of anxiety

Nursing diagnosis	• For parents/guardians the risk of anxiety is related to knowledge deficit about the surgery and its outcomes
Expected outcome	• No anxiety
Nursing intervention and rationale	• Provide information and explain the pathology of the defect, manifestations, the possible prognosis and various modalities of care and treatment to the parents. Point out potential problems such as strictures to parents/guardians

	• Support parents/guardians as needed. Encourage them to cuddle and hold the child frequently, as bonding at birth might have been disrupted by the need for emergency care
• Encourage parents/guardians to participate in the care of the child. This helps them learn how to care for the child at home after discharge
• Refer parents/guardians to a physiotherapist for assistance with prescribed exercises
• Teach parents/guardians how to observe for strictures, which may be a late complication. Signs for strictures are choking or gagging on solid food, increased drooling, dysphagia and frequent coughing and choking related to swallowing
• Encourage the parents/guardians to talk about the child's condition. Allow them to ask questions and to express their fears and concerns freely. If parents can accept the situation they are likely to participate in the care much more willingly than they otherwise would
• Provide counselling for parents/guardians and refer them to a psychologist for further professional counselling if this is deemed necessary.
Evaluation	• Parents are able to talk about the child's condition freely and are participating in the care

Conclusion

Oesophageal atresia and trachea-oesophageal fistula may occur separately or together. In all instances, they are an emergency. The nurse in the labour ward must treat newborns who have respiratory diseases at birth as having an abnormality relating to oesophogeal atresia with or without tracheal fistula until proven otherwise. This will allow for emergency treatment that helps save many lives.

Congenital diaphragmatic hernia

The diaphragm is a muscle that separates the thoracic cavity from the abdominal cavity. It assists with respiration, whereby its contraction increases the thoracic cavity, allowing the lungs to expand during inspiration and its relaxation decreases the thoracic cavity, allowing for expiration. Congenital diaphragmatic hernia is a birth defect where there is failure of the pleuro-peritoneal outgrowths of the lateral and posterior thoracic cavity to fuse during embryonic development

Pathophysiology. The diaphragm is formed from the 4th to the 8th week of gestation. Diaphragmatic hernia is as a result of failure of the pleuro-peritoneal outgrowths to fuse. It is marked by a weakness in the continuity of the diaphragm or an abnormal opening in the continuity of the diaphragm posteriorly, whereby the contents of the abdominal cavity may herniate into the thoracic cavity. The herniation can occur during foetal development or at birth. If the herniation occurs during foetal development, the lung development is compromised, giving rise to a condition known as lung hypoplasia.

Clinical manifestations
- There may be a history of polyhydramnios during the pregnancy and prematurity at birth.
- The child has a scaphoid abdomen, which is an indication that the abdominal contents may have moved into the thoracic cavity, leaving the abdominal cavity empty or the abdomen area hollow.
- At birth, the child has acute respiratory distress and cyanosis. The APGAR score is low. This is an indication that the abdominal contents that have escaped into the thoracic cavity are pressing onto the lungs and the large blood vessels.
- There may be signs and symptoms of shock where blood vessels are also compressed.

Assessment findings

Three diagnostic signs are polyhydramnios, mediastinal shift seen on X-ray, and loops of bowel are seen in the thoracic cavity. The diagnosis can be done prenatally and the advantage of this is that the parents can be counselled on pregnancy alternatives and potential problems of the neonatal period. Furthermore, the attending antenatal care team is able to prepare for the management of this neonate at birth.

At birth, the diagnosis is done based on clinical manifestations and confirmed with the chest X-ray.

Management of congenital diaphragmatic hernia

This is an emergency which carries a high mortality. The child must be resuscitated with care so as not to inflate the lungs, as these are compressed. The child is transferred to the intensive care unit.

Nursing management

A child diagnosed with congenital diaphragmatic hernia must be prepared for surgery in the following way:
- Keep the child warm to avoid hypothermia. Ideally the child is nursed in an incubator.
- A nasogastric tube is inserted to deflate the stomach, which may be located in the thoracic cavity.
- The child is weighed, so that medication dosages and fluid requirements can be calculated.
- A pulse oximeter may be clipped on to the finger to monitor oxygen saturation.
- Temperature, pulse and respiration are monitored, especially where there is respiratory distress.
- The child is put in a high-Fowler's position to try to get the abdominal contents back into the abdominal cavity by gravity.
- An intravenous infusion for glucose and electrolytes is put up to prevent hypoglycaemia and electrolyte imbalance and an intake-and-output record is kept.

Postoperative care

Post-operatively the child will have a nasogastric tube to decompress the stomach, and intravenous infusion and transfusion lines for fluids and blood. There may be a wound drain as well. The care includes:

- Routine observations to ensure that:
  - the intravenous infusion and transfusion are flowing as prescribed to prevent fluid imbalances and shock
  - the nasogastric tube is draining
  - the wound drain is working
  - the temperature is monitored every 15 minutes to prevent hypothermia and to detect and treat infection early if present
  - the child should be monitored for respiratory distress
- Care should be taken to keep the child's skin clean and dry. The child will be sedated for long periods of time, so their position needs to be changed periodically and parents/guardians assisted to hold the child on their lap as a measure to relieve pressure on the skin.
- Pain should be managed as prescribed.
- Feeding should be commenced as soon as the child is stable and bowel sounds are heard.
- Also see Table 7.3.

Table 7.3: Specific postoperative nursing care plan of a child who has undergone repair of congenital diaphragmatic hernia

Problem: Pain	
Nursing diagnosis	• Altered comfort due to pain related to surgery performed, evidenced by restlessness, crying and pallor
Expected outcome	• Relieve pain and discomfort
Nursing intervention and rationale	• Assess pain adequately to get baseline data against which to measure progress • Administer analgesics as prescribed to relieve pain. • Ensure that no lines are blocked, as these may cause pain if not draining or running well, eg drips should not infiltrate • Prevent hypothermia. Nurse in an incubator or cover the patient lightly to ensure correct and comfortable temperature • Engage the physiotherapist to help with respiration to expand the lung that might have collapsed or help develop the hypoplastic lung that was compressed by the abdominal contents • Help the patient to assume a comfortable position without stretching the incision or pressing on it. This may be a high-Fowler's position to help the abdominal contents return to the abdominal cavity by gravity • Monitor and record vital signs to identify haemorrhage and infection, which could be the cause of pain and discomfort.
Evaluation	• Child is sleeping peacefully and responding to sedation. No crying

Problem: Respiratory distress	
Nursing diagnosis	• Altered breathing related to the surgical condition and the treatment thereof
Expected outcome	• Child breathing with ease
Nursing intervention and rationale	• Put the child in a high-Fowler's position, if permitted, to allow for the abdominal contents to return to the abdominal cavity by gravity
• Ensure that the underwater seal drainage is draining and functioning well to assist with the expansion of the lung.
• Monitor oxygen as prescribed
• Monitor vital signs quarter-hourly to detect progress in the improvement of breathing as well as to enable the early detection and treatment of infection, if suspected
• Record any cyanotic attacks, as these dictate the degree of respiratory distress experienced
• Engage a physiotherapist for passive exercises to help with lung expansion and improved air intake.
Evaluation	• Respiratory rate within normal range, indicating improved expansion of the lung. No cyanotic attacks. Vital signs normal as there would be no infection
Problem: Risk of infection	
Nursing diagnosis	• Risk of wound infection related to surgery
• Risk of lung infection (prostatic pneumonia) related to atelectasis following compression by abdominal contents.
Expected outcome	• Prevent and minimise wound and lung infection
Nursing intervention and rationale	• Monitor vital signs and take note and report increased breathing rate and rhythm
• Administer and record analgesics and antibiotics as prescribed
• Maintain asepsis when attending to the wound and report any bleeding, pain and inflammation
• Apply dressing to support the wound
• Monitor and record intravenous infusion to prevent dehydration
• Provide breast milk or formula feed in a bottle with a large hole to reduce the sucking effort. The breast milk or formula has the necessary nutrients to support tissue growth and therefore wound healing.
Evaluation	• Get the parent/guardian to hold the child on their lap as soon as is permitted as a way of getting them out of bed early. This might also serve as exercise to improve circulation as well as a way to calm the child down

Problem: Hydration and nutrition	
Nursing diagnosis	• Fluid volume deficit and altered nutrition related to preoperative care, which requires that the child takes nothing orally, and the nasogastric suctioning pre- and postoperatively
Expected outcome	• Maintain normal hydration and normal nutrition
Nursing intervention and rationale	• Monitor the intravenous line and administer intravenous fluids as prescribed to maintain hydration. Record fluid intake
• Ensure that the nasogastric tube is draining and record the drainage as fluid output. Leave the nasogastric tube in situ until bowel sounds are heard and the child is stable
• Start the intake of oral fluids with small sips and amounts of clear water, followed by expressed breast milk or formula feed
• Increase the feeds gradually to avoid sudden distension of the stomach.
Evaluation	• The child is well-hydrated and gaining weight as expected
Problem: Risk of anxiety	
Nursing diagnosis	• For the parents/guardians, the risk of anxiety is related to knowledge deficit about the surgery and its outcomes
Expected outcome	• No anxiety for the parents/guardians
Nursing intervention and rationale	• Provide information and explain the disease pathology, causes, manifestations, possible prognosis and possible modalities of care and treatment to parents/guardians
• Provide information about available alternatives to treatment
• Refer to physiotherapy to assist with the prescribed exercises
• Encourage the parents/guardians to talk about the child's condition and allow them to ask questions and to verbalise fears and concerns freely. If parents/guardians can accept the situation, they are more likely to participate in the care than they otherwise might be
• Provide counselling for parents/guardians and refer them to the psychologist for further professional counselling if this is deemed necessary.
Evaluation	• Parents are able to talk about the child's condition freely and are participating in the care

Conclusion

Congenital diaphragmatic hernia is a very frightening conditionforto parents, as the child is usually desperately ill immediately after birth. The complicated operation that needs to be done is also difficult for parents to understand. As in many other cases of congenital defects parents might blame themselves for the plight of their child. This self-blame makes it even more difficult for parents to accept the situation.

Hypertrophic pyloric stenosis

The pylorus is that part of the gastrointestinal tract that links the stomach to the duodenum. It is a sphincter that prevents the back flow of gastric contents once they have been pushed into the duodenum (see Figure 7.2).

Pathophysiology. Pyloric stenosis is result of progressive hypertrophy of the circular sphincter muscle of the pylorus progressively narrowing the pyloric canal to the point of obstructing the pyloric outlet.

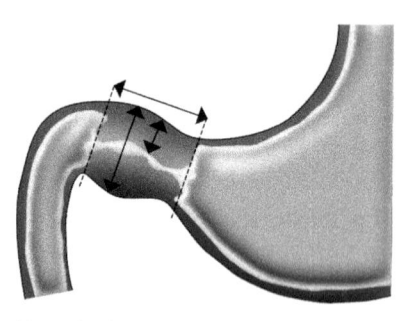

Normal values
Length: <15 mm
Single thickness: <3 mm
Pyloric width: <7 mm

Figure 7.2 Pyloric stenosis

The cause of this hypertrophy is not known, but is linked to genetic factors. There is a higher incidence in children with a previous family history of pyloric stenosis. It is more common in first-born children and in boys rather than in girls.

Clinical manifestations

The signs are progressive, whereby in the 2nd week after birth the child will regurgitate much more feed than is usual. The child is irritable and always hungry, as most of the feed is regurgitated and they may fail to thrive. There may be dehydration if this is not corrected, as it will progress to non-projectile vomiting after feeding. Projectile vomiting may happen in the 4th week when the canal is totally obstructed. Projectile vomiting is sudden and peristalsis pre-obstruction is strong and visible as gastric contents are trying to push through the obstruction. The hypertrophic muscles are palpable and sometimes visible as a mass at the point of the obstruction.

7.1 Defining signs of hypertrophic pyloric stenosis include:

- Characteristic projectile vomiting, which is
  - vomitus ejected from the child
  - vomiting not preceded by retching and occurring after a feed
  - vomitus that consists of fresh or curdled milk – the vomitus does not contain bile and will turn blue litmus paper red because it is acidic in nature.
- The child:
  - is always hungry and feeding eagerly, only to vomit after the feed
  - fails to thrive and may show signs of dehydration
  - has a distended abdomen pre-obstruction
  - displays visible peristalsis across the epigastrium from left to right
  - has a palpable mass in the epigastrium
  - is constipated (is not passing stools).

Management
The hypertrophy is usually relieved surgically by a procedure called pyloromyotomy or Ramstedt's procedure during which the hypertrophied circular muscles are incised down to the submucosa lining of the gut. The procedure has a high success rate.

Specific preoperative care
In the preoperative care of a child with hypertrophy, they must be kept nil per os with a nasogastric tube inserted to decompress the dilated stomach. Specific steps for preoperative care are as follows:
- The child is weighed for the calculation of fluids and medication.
- Hypothermia is prevented by adequate covering of the child.
- The intravenous infusion therapy of dextrose and electrolytes is monitored and maintained to correct hydration and electrolyte imbalance.
- An accurate description of vomiting (its nature, amount, frequency) and that of faecal elimination by the child is kept.
- An accurate record of intake and output is kept.

Where there is no evidence of fluid and electrolyte imbalance, the operation is done as soon as the diagnosis is made, otherwise it can be delayed for 24 hours to correct the fluid and electrolyte imbalances.

For perioperative care, refer to Chapters 3, 4 and 5.

Specific postoperative care
Observations that were made preoperatively are continued postoperatively. These include:
- Observe for any continued vomiting in the first 24 to 48 hours. This could be due to the partial relaxation of the hypertrophied muscles, which will stabilise with time. A record of the nature, amount and frequency of the vomiting is kept.
- The nasogastric tube is left in situ until there is no drainage reported and bowel sounds are heard. A record of drainage is kept.

- The intravenous therapy is maintained and monitored.
- Analgesics are administered for pain as prescribed.
- Vital signs are monitored and any changes are recorded and reported.
- The operated site is observed for any bleeding, exudate or inflammation.
- Feeding is commenced within 6 to 8 hours postoperatively, provided there are bowel sounds and the child is not vomiting. At first the child is given small amounts of water and, if this is retained, small amounts of milk feed are given at frequent intervals. If the child is breastfed, the mother is supervised on how to breastfeed.
The child is usually discharged from hospital within 5 to 7 days.

Intussusception

This is not a congenital condition and it occurs commonly when the child is introduced to solids around 9 months to a year. It can also happen at any time in the first 6 years and at any site in the intestines and the colon.

Pathophysiology. Intussusception refers to the invagination or telescoping of the proximal segment of the bowel into a more distal segment pulling the mesentery with it. There is a risk of obstruction of blood and lymph vessels that supply the affected mesentery and the bowel (see Figure 7.3 below). The result of the obstruction of arterial supply is ischaemia, while that of the veins and lymph vessels is engorgement, which results in the leaking of blood and mucus into the intestinal lumen, forming the characteristic 'red currant jelly' like stool. The most common site is at the ileocaecal valve, where the ileum invaginates into the caecum.

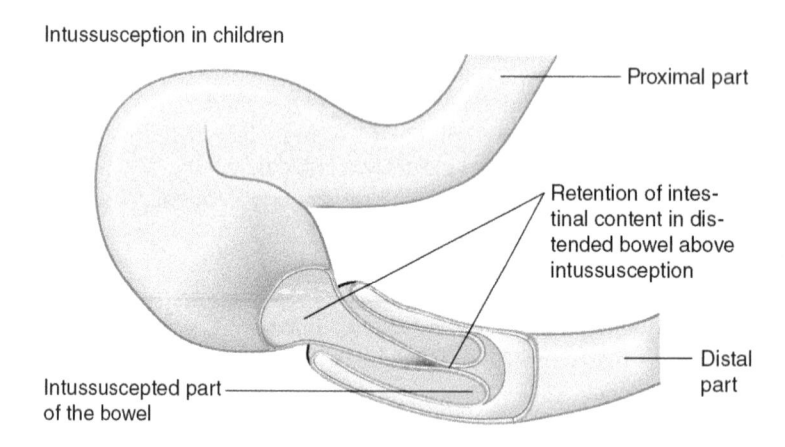

Figure 7.3 Intussusception in children

Types of intussusception
There are three types of intussusception. They are explained as follows:
- **Ileocaecal.** The ileum invaginates into the caecum (see Figure 7.4).
- **Ileoileal.** A part of the ileum invaginates into the adjacent section of the ileum.
- **Colocolonic.** One part of the colon invaginates into another adjacent area of the colon.

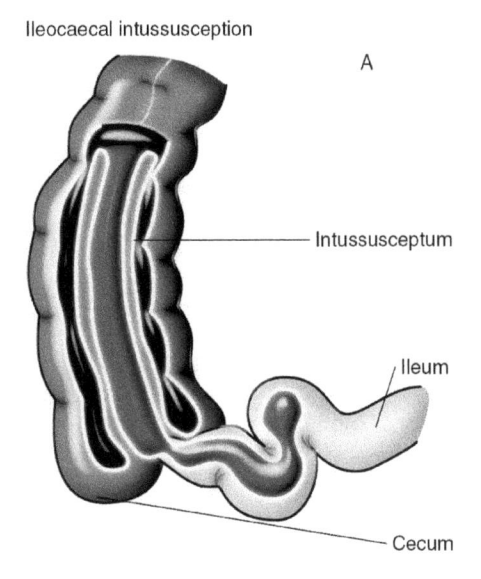

Figure 7.4 Ileocaecal intussusception

Clinical manifestations
- Child becomes flushed and cries at the sudden onset of colicky abdominal pain. The child's knees are drawn up to their chest.
- The pain comes in intervals and each time it comes with renewed intensity pain is synchronised with peristalsis.
- The child is constipated but may pass a small blood-stained mucoid stool ('red currant jelly' stool).
- On palpation, a mass may be felt over the place of invagination.

Assessment findings
Subjective data
The nurse can help confirm the diagnosis from the parent's/guardian's description of the signs and symptoms. Characteristic signs include the typical abdominal pain, abdominal mass and blood-stained mucoid stool. Vomiting may be present with the progression of obstruction.

Management of intussusception
Management of intussusception is surgical in nature, where upon the intussusception can be reduced with the use of a contrast enema. Where ischaemia has resulted in gangrene of the bowel, the gangrenous bowel is resected and the healthy bowel ends are anastomosed.

Specific preoperative care
Once the diagnosis is made, a mode of management is decided upon. The operative care entails the usual care for all abdominal surgery, which includes the following:
- continued observation of the stool
- positioning the child in an upright position to facilitate self-resolution

- monitoring and maintaining intravenous infusion therapy
- inserting a nasogastric tube to decompress the abdomen and reduce the risk of vomiting
- monitoring the vital signs
- keeping the child warm
- administering antibiotics as prescribed for a gangrenous bowel

> **Clinical alert!**
> Passage of a normal stool may be an indication that the intussusception has reduced itself and the operation may be unnecessary.

Specific postoperative care
This is the same as for all abdominal surgical procedures. It includes monitoring of the IV line, nasogastric tube drainage, wound drainage and observation of wound dressings, and recording of all the observations. Monitoring of the vital signs remain crucial to identify infection early for early management. An upright position is maintained to facilitate or maintain a disentangled gut. Administration of antibiotics as prescribed is also important, especially in cases where the bowel may be gangrenous.

Potential postoperative care problems
Infection. Peritonitis is a risk, especially where there was ischaemia and gangrene in the bowel.
Paralytic ileus. May result from overhandling of the intestines and bowel when the intussusception is released.
Recurrence of the intussusception. Occurs especially where the reduction was spontaneous or with the use of an enema.

Volvulus
Volvulus is a serious type of intestinal obstruction (see Figures 7.5 (a) A to C)). It can be congenital or acquired. If congenital, it is referred to as malrotation. It is a defect that occurs in the midgut where the intestines fail to differentiate or rotate correctly. If acquired, the intestine twists around itself, thus compromising blood supply, which results in intestinal necrosis, peritonitis, perforation and death.

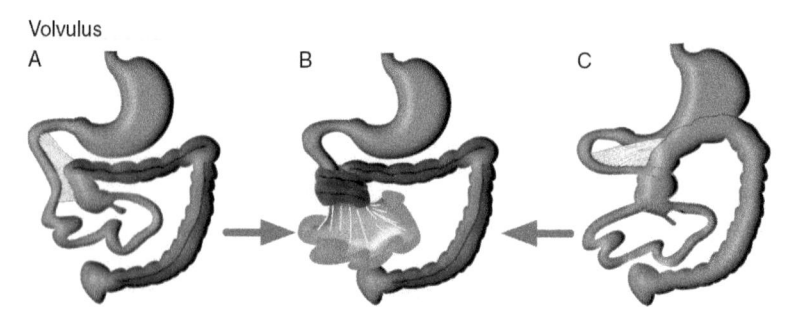

Figure 7.5 (a) Volvulus

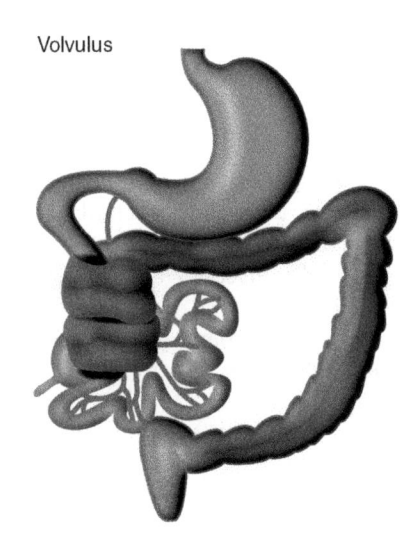

Figure 7.5 (b) Volvulus

Clinical manifestation
The child will present with all the signs of intestinal obstruction:
- abdominal colicky pain made worse by peristalsis
- there may be vomiting
- abdominal distension with constipation
- dehydration.

Specific preoperative care
This will be the same as that provided for other intestinal obstruction: IV therapy maintenance and monitoring to correct dehydration and electrolyte imbalances, a nasogastric tube is inserted to decompress abdominal distension, vital signs are monitored to exclude infection (peritonitis), adequate cover to prevent hypothermia, and positioning the child in an upright position.

Surgical management includes the correction of the rotation where possible, resection of necrosed portions and anastomosis of the healthy parts to form continuity of the gut.

Specific postoperative care
This is the same as that provided for abdominal surgery to relieve intestinal obstruction. It includes monitoring and maintenance of IV lines, a nasogastric tube is inserted to drain gastric contents and relieve gastric distension and the administration of antibiotics.

Congenital aganglionic megacolon (Hirschsprung's disease)
Congenital aganglionic megacolon is a defect that arises from lack of innervation in a segment of the hindgut during embryonic development. The hindgut is that portion of the embryonic gut that forms the proximal two thirds of the transverse colon, the descending colon, sigmoid colon, the rectum and the anal canal. In aganglionic megacolon there is an absence of autonomic parasympathetic ganglion cells of the mysenteric and submucous plexuses that innervate a portion of the colon, resulting in poor or no peristalsis in the

affected portion. The affected portion is usually small and it therefore takes time for the signs to manifest (see Figure 7.6).

Clinical manifestations

These may vary from chronic constipation to acute mechanical obstruction. Meconium is passed in the first 24 to 36 hours after birth. In children suspected with aganglionic megacolon there may be a delay or failure to pass meconium at birth after the mandatory 36 hours. Affected children might also present with vomiting and abdominal distension. Older children might present with a history of alternating constipation and bouts of diarrhoea and abdominal distension with vomiting. With constipation the stool is like flat pellets. In some instances, the vomitus may be bile-stained or faecal-smelling. The child fails to thrive, and is malnourished.

The abdomen is distended and, on rectal examination, the rectum is often empty of stool.

Objective data to confirm diagnosis includes a rectal biopsy, an X-ray and a barium enema, which will demonstrate the transition between the agangliotic segment and the distended megacolon segment.

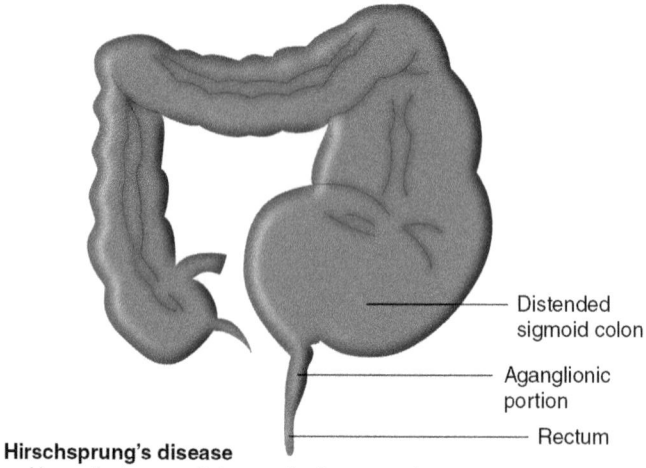

Hirschsprung's disease
- Also called congenital aganglionic megacolon
- Mechanical obstruction from inadequate motility of the intestine
- Incidence: 1 in 5 000 live births; more common in males and in children with Down syndrome
- Absence of ganglion cells in colon

Figure 7.6 Aganglionic megacolon with significant presentations

Surgical management is done in stages and may include resection of the agangliotic segment and a colostomy that can be temporary or permanent depending on the child's response to the initial surgery.

Specific preoperative care
Preoperative care involves extensive cleaning of the bowel with enemata and bowel washout, as well as:
- an assessment of the nutrition and hydration status of the child and the monitoring of serum electrolytes. This will require blood tests and other related tests such as a rectal biopsy and a barium enema
- monitored intravenous infusion therapy
- parental education as a form of preoperative care. Parents/guardians must be informed on the use of enemata and aperients such as purgatives and laxatives. If enemas are required at home these should be isotonic saline enemata. Parents/guardians are given instructions on how to administer these. Parents also need to be trained stoma care in the event of a colostomy.

Specific postoperative care
Postoperative care is the same as for all other abdominal procedures, as is indicated below:
- The nasogastric tube is kept in situ until bowel sounds are heard.
- Oral feeds are withheld while the nasogastric tube is in situ.
- Intravenous infusion therapy provides fluids and electrolytes.
- Stoma care is provided.
- Parents/guardians are given instructions and demonstrations on stoma care, and the child is not discharged from the hospital until parents/guardians are confident about stoma care. Information and details of contact persons are given to them should they need help with stoma care and stoma appliances.
- Home care follow-up may be provided by the stoma therapist on request.

Imperforate anus
Imperforate anus is a term used to address a group of anorectal malformations. The anus and rectum develop from the embryonic hindgut. The development is usually complete by the 8th week of gestation and anything that interrupts the process may result in anorectal malformations. The anus may be stenosed, closed or absent. The rectum may end in a blind pouch either below or above the levator ani muscle. A fistula may also exist between the anorectal structures and the perineum, urethra, bladder or vagina.

Clinical manifestations
At birth, the child may be unable to pass meconium or pass a ribbon-like stool indicating some form of stenosis. The nurse may be unable to pass a finger through during physical examination or the rectal thermometer may not be able to pass through to measure vital statistics for baseline data.

In some instances, anorectal deformities may only be apparent later when the child presents with chronic constipation.

Assessment and common findings
Infants suspected of anorectal malformations must be examined thoroughly to establish other related anomalies of the pelvis and vertebrae as well as fistulae linking the structures with the perineum, bladder, urethra and vagina.

The nurse is usually the first person to discover anorectal anomalies during temperature taking. In their observations they may notice that the child has not passed meconium in the first 24 hours and the abdomen might be distended.

Management
This is determined by the position of the defect. The operations are usually done in stages, with the aim to assist the child to achieve continence without problems.

For pre- and intraoperative care, see Chapters 3, 4 and 5.

Specific postoperative care
In hospital, postoperative care includes the prevention of infection and providing information to alleviate anxiety. When the child is ready to be discharged, it is important that the family is taught manual dilatation for anal stenosis, which can be done at home. Parents need to know that children with anorectal deformities may have difficulties with toilet training, therefore they need to be patient and persistent in establishing a daily routine for elimination. Young children may need to be encouraged to use the toilet after every feed to avoid soiling themselves. In terms of nutrition and hydration, the child must take adequate fluids and follow a high-fibre diet. Some children may need stool softeners to avoid stool impaction.

Hernias
A hernia is a protrusion of a portion of an organ or organs through an abnormal opening. In some instances, it can be incarcerated or strangulated. An incarcerated hernia cannot be reduced manually but there is no interference with blood supply. A strangulated hernia is a protrusion where an opening is small and there is interference with the blood supply to the protruding portion to the extent that the protruding part can be ischaemic.

Types of hernias
- Omphalocele
- Umbilical hernia
- Inguinal hernia
- Diaphragmatic hernia

Omphalocele
Pathophysiology. An omphalocele is a congenital defect where the intestines herniate into the umbilical cord and fail to return to the abdominal cavity by the 10th week of gestation during the embryonic stage due to a defective abdominal wall next to the umbilicus. The intestines are covered by the amniotic membrane. The defect, although rare, is associated with other defects such, as Meckel diverticulum and trisomy 13. The omphalocele is a precursor to volvulus, as intestines that fail to re-enter the abdominal cavity may become malrotated.

Clinical manifestations. The intestines that are outside the abdominal cavity may be oedematous at birth, presenting with obstruction. The amniotic sac may rupture, which may lead to infection.

Potential problems resulting from an omphalocele are:
- infection if the membrane ruptures, which may result in septicaemia.
- loss of heat and fluids, depending on the extent of the area exposed in the rupture
- intestinal obstruction and/or infarction may be present if herniation is incarcerated, as this may result in oedema.

Specific preoperative care:
- Cover the exposed intestine with a warm, sterile saline dressing to prevent hypothermia.
- Nurse the child in isolation in an incubator to keep the baby warm.
- Assess for signs of infection by monitoring vital signs.
- Maintain intravenous infusion for dextrose and electrolytes.
- Provide counselling to parents/guardians.

Specific postoperative care
To prevent infection:
- the child is nursed in isolation in an incubator that keeps them warm to prevent hypothermia
- wound care is done aseptically.

Hydration and nutrition:
- Maintain intravenous infusion for dextrose and electrolytes.
- Monitor the child's nutrition, because the bowel might be resected and the baby may require parenteral nutrition until the feeding is stable.
- Monitor the child's growth, as nutrition may be compromised.

Potential for injury:
- Minimise the child's movements by giving prescribed analgesics to control pain.

Parental anxiety:
- Anxiety in parents/guardians may be due to knowledge deficit. Provide as much information as is possible about the condition, its possible causes, planned management and what the parents'/guardians' contribution could be. Refer them for counselling if necessary.

Umbilical hernia
Umbilical hernia is the protrusion of part of the intestines through the abdominal wall at the umbilical ring when the fusion was incomplete at the point where the umbilical vessels exit the abdominal wall. The size of the defect is variable and the protrusion is more prominent during crying. Nursing management of a child with umbilical hernia includes reassurance of the parents.
Clinical manifestation. Umbilical hernia presents as a soft, reducible swelling at the umbilicus, covered by the peritoneum and the skin. The hernia regresses spontaneously.

Inguinal hernia

Pathophysiology. Inguinal hernia results from the persistence of the processus vaginalis, the tube of peritoneum that precedes the testicle through the inguinal canal into the scrotum (in males) or the round ligament into the labia (in females) during the 8th month of gestation. Normally, after the descent of the testicle, the proximal portion of the processus vaginalis atrophies and closes, whereas the distal portion forms the tunica vaginalis, which encases the testicle. When the upper portion fails to close, some abdominal and pelvic structures (small intestine), ovary or fallopian tube) may slip down into the inguinal canal, through the external ring and into the scrotum, creating a palpable bulge or mass. Management of inguinal hernias is surgical and, in uncomplicated presentations, it is elective.

Clinical manifestations. There is usually a painless inguinal lump. This lump may disappear at times of relaxation or can be reduced or pushed back manually by gentle compression. The lump appears when the child cries, strains, coughs or stands for a long time. The defect can be traced as a thick cord in the groin.

Invariably, if the bowel herniates into the inguinal canal, there may be signs of obstruction and others such as constipation, irritability, anorexia, tenderness and abdominal distension. The bowel may be incarcerated or strangulated, with signs and symptoms of complete intestinal obstruction. Should the obstruction not be corrected, the strangulated bowel may become gangrenous and necrotic.

Specific preoperative care

There is no specific preoperative care for the repair of aninguinal hernia. This is usually an elective type of surgery. For preoperative care, refer to Chapters 3, 4 and 5.

The child is admitted the day before the operation for blood tests and X-rays if these were not done during clinic visits. The parents/guardians are counselled and given information about the operation and an informed consent is sought. The anaesthetist and the theatre nurse have to assess the child to confirm readiness for surgery.

Specific postoperative care

This includes:
- pain management: analgesics are administered as prescribed
- wound care: aseptic technique to be maintained in wound care
- positioning the child comfortably and avoiding positions that elicit discomfort
- observations for:
  - haemorrhage: monitor vital signs. Vital signs are monitored every quarter of an hour for the first 6 hours, and every 30 minutes for the next 6 hours. If stable, these are monitored 4-hourly after 12 hours. This is to identify any internal haemorrhage as indicated by a thready pulse, restlessness and pallor. If present, report to the surgeon and record for reference
  - infection: observe any bleeding of the wound. This is very important, especially 24 hours post-surgery when the bleeding could be secondary to infection. Monitor vital signs as stated above. A body temperature above 38 °C must be reported, as this could be an indication of infection. Pain and swelling must also be reported

Table 7.4 A general postoperative nursing care plan for a child who has undergone surgery of the intestines or repair of inguinal hernia

Problem: Pain	
Nursing diagnosis	• Altered comfort due to pain related to surgery, evidenced by restlessness, crying and pallor, and if child is old enough, verbal expression of pain
Expected outcome	• No discomfort or pain
Nursing intervention and rationale	• Assess pain adequately to get baseline data against which to measure progress
• Administer analgesics as prescribed to relieve pain.
• Ensure that no lines are blocked, as these may cause pain if not draining or running well, eg drips should not infiltrate, catheters should flow, and wound drains should drain the blood away from the wound to effect proper circulation and reduce oedema
• Maintain body temperature and prevent hypothermia. Cover the patient lightly to ensure correct and comfortable temperature. An incubator is used for newborns
• Help the patient to assume a comfortable position without stretching the incision or pressing on it. This may be a high-Fowler's position to help with the expansion of the lungs and to expose the incision. Change the patient's position from side to side and side to recumbent to facilitate circulation and promote comfort further
• Engage a physiotherapist to help with respiration to expand the lungs further, and to support the incision during coughing and breathing exercises
• Monitor and record vital signs to identify increasing pulse and respiratory rates in particular, as pain and discomfort might be an indicator for haemorrhage and infection
Evaluation	• Child is sleeping peacefully and responding to sedation. There is no restlessness and crying
Problem: Risk of haemorrhage	
Nursing diagnosis	• Risk of fluid volume deficit related to bleeding postoperatively is evidenced by restlessness, pallor and a thready pulse
Expected outcome	• Child maintains hydration. There is no haemorrhage
Nursing intervention and rationale	• Monitor and record vital signs hourly for 12 hours, and if child is stable, increase the observation time to 2-hourly for the next 12 hours, so that changes can be detected and managed early. If child remains stable, vital signs can be monitored every 4 hours
• Observe the wound site and dressings for any bleeding. If bleeding is observed, report this to the surgeon immediately while you pack the wound

	• Administer volume expanders, blood and blood products as prescribed
	• Administer and record intravenous fluids and electrolytes as prescribed to prevent dehydration and electrolyte imbalance, which can compromise wound healing
	• Monitor and record urinary output and stools and all other outputs such as vomitus, blood loss and insensible loss, so that replacement is estimated correctly to avoid fluid overload.
Evaluation	• There is no bleeding. Vital signs are normal

Problem: Risk of infection

Nursing diagnosis	• Risk of wound infection related to surgery
	• Risk of lung infection (prostatic and aspiration pneumonia) related to immobility and vomiting
	• Risk of peritonitis.
Expected outcome	• No wound and lung infection, no peritonitis
Nursing intervention and rationale	• Monitor vital signs and take note of and report increased breathing rate and rhythm, and increased temperature.
	• Administer and record analgesics and antibiotics as prescribed
	• Maintain asepsis when attending to the wound and report any bleeding, pain and inflammation
	• Apply dressing to support the wound
	• Monitor and record intravenous infusion to prevent dehydration
	• Provide breast milk or formula feed in a bottle with a big hole to reduce the sucking effort. Breast milk or formula has the necessary nutrients to support tissue growth and therefore wound healing. For older children, provide a nutritious diet rich in proteins, minerals and vitamins to support tissue repair and growth
	• Engage a physiotherapist to assist the patient with breathing and coughing exercises to help expectorate secretions from the lungs
	• Put the child in the most comfortable position and change the child's position every 2 hours to loosen the lung secretions
	• Get the parents/guardians to hold the child in their lap as soon as is permitted as a way of getting the child out of bed early to improve circulation. This might also serve as exercise to improve circulation and as a way to calm the child down
	• Observe the abdomen for distension and the child's general condition to exclude peritonitis. Listen for bowel sounds and do not commence with feeds if bowel sounds are not audible. If a nasogastric tube was inserted postoperatively, this is left in situ to drain until bowel sounds are heard

Evaluation	• Vital signs are normal. Child is comfortable and feeding well
Problem: Risk of paralytic ileus	
Nursing diagnosis	• Altered comfort due to abdominal distension and pain related to surgery and anaesthesia
Expected outcome	• No abdominal distension and no pain
Nursing intervention and rationale	• Ensure that the nasogastric tube is in situ and draining. Patients who have had intestinal surgery are at risk of paralytic ileus, and the draining nasogastric tube will ensure that the stomach is empty, that peristalsis is kept to a minimum and that the gut can rest until muscle tone returns
• Patient should not be given anything orally postoperatively until bowel sounds are heard and the patient is passing flatus. At this stage small amounts of clear fluids should be given until tolerated, followed by small amounts of breast milk, formula or solids (soft diet). Normal amounts of food or feeds should be given when tolerance of small amounts of oral feeds or food is confirmed
• If there is abdominal distension, abdominal girth should be measured and recorded daily. The nasogastric tube should be left to drain
• Encourage the parents/guardians to hold the child in their lap. Change the child's position 2-hourly and if the child can walk help the child to take a few steps out of bed. This will stimulate peristalsis and improve muscle tone
• Reduce pain by supporting the operated site with bandages, and give non-constipating analgesics because pain may cause immobility, which may cause constipation.
Evaluation	• Bowel sounds are heard. Patient passes flatus.
Problem: Hydration and nutrition	
Nursing diagnosis	• Risk of fluid volume deficit and altered nutrition lower than body requirements related to preoperative care, which requires that the child takes nothing orally, and nasogastric suctioning pre- and postoperatively
Expected outcome	• Child maintains normal hydration and normal nutrition and gains weight as an indication of normal growth

Nursing intervention and rationale	• Monitor the intravenous line and administer intravenous fluids as prescribed to maintain hydration. Record fluid intake and output • Ensure that the nasogastric tube is draining and record the drainage as fluid output. Leave the nasogastric tube in situ until certain that there is no vomiting, bowel sounds are heard and the child is stable • If bowel sounds are heard, start the intake of oral fluids with small sips of clear water, followed by expressed breast milk or formula once the child tolerates water. Follow up the clear fluids/water with very small amounts of soft diet • Increase the feeds gradually to avoid sudden distension of the stomach • Weigh the child daily to assess weight gain and general growth and record in graph form
Evaluation	• Child is well-hydrated and gaining weight as expected
Problem: Risk of anxiety	
Nursing diagnosis	• For parent/guardians the risk of anxiety related to knowledge deficit about the surgery and its outcomes
Expected outcome	• No anxiety
Nursing intervention and rationale	• Provide information and explain the pathophysiology of the disease, manifestations, possible prognosis and possible modalities of care and treatment to parents/guardians • Provide information to parents/guardian about available alternatives to treatment and how parents/guardians can participate in these treatments • Refer parents/guardians to a physiotherapist to assist with the prescribed exercises • Encourage parents to talk about the child's condition and allow them to ask questions and to verbalise fears and concerns freely. If parents can accept the situation they are likely to participate in the care much more willing than they otherwise would • Provide counselling for parents/guardians and refer them to a psychologist for further professional counselling if needed
Evaluation	• Parents able to talk about the child's condition freely and are participating in the care

Conclusion

Intestinal surgery to correct conditions indicated in this chapter is common in general paediatric wards. General nurses therefore need to know how children presenting with these conditions are cared for before, during and after surgery. It is critical for nurses to ensure that the child's gut is empty preoperatively to prevent vomiting during and after surgery. The intraoperative safety of the child is critical. Always ensure that the correct child is being operated by checking the patient's name, age, hospital registration, diagnosis and operation site. Safety also relates to prevention of falls, correct dosage of medication and maintaining the correct temperature. Postoperatively, it is critical to monitor and record the patient's vital signs, as these are reliable indicators of potential problems.

Suggested activities for learners

Activity 7.1
1. Explain how you would counsel a mother who has just given birth to a child with a diaphragmatic hernia to convince her to give consent for the repair of the hernia.
2. Discuss any three potential risks that exist with the postoperative repair of the diaphragmatic hernia.
3. Explain (with illustrations) the different types of oesophageal and tracheal anomalies and associated potential problems.
4. Indicate the potential risks for a child with oesophageal atresia with a tracheal fistula.
5. Explain the preoperative care of a child diagnosed with a trachea-oesophageal fistula and provide reasons for activities undertaken.
6. What is the difference between an incarcerated hernia and a strangulated hernia? What are the implications of both?

Reference

Hockenberry, MJ, & Wilson, D. 2015. *Wong's nursing care of infants and children*. 10th edition. Elsevier.

Mogotlane, S, Mokoena, J, Chauke, M, Matlakala, M, Young, A, & Randa, B. 2018. *Juta's complete textbook of medical surgical nursing*. 2nd edition. Cape Town: Juta.

Mott, SR, James, SR, & Sperhac, AM. 1990. *Nursing care of children and families*. 2nd edition. New York: Addison-Wesley Nursing.

Skandalakis, JE, & Gray, SW. 1994. *Embryology for surgeons: the embryological basis for the treatment of congenital anomalies*. 2nd edition. Baltimore: Williams & Wilkins.

Section 4

Inflammatory surgical conditions

8 Acute appendicitis and appendicectomy

LEARNING OBJECTIVES

On completion of this Chapter, you should be able to:
- describe the causes, pathophysiology and clinical manifestations of appendicitis in child care
- describe the assessment of a child diagnosed with appendicitis
- explain the nursing management of a child with appendicitis for appendicectomy.

KEY CONCEPTS AND TERMINOLOGY	
adhesions:	These are areas in the gastrointestinal tract that stick together or stick on to other parts of the intestines, causing obstruction in the intestinal lumen.
anorexia:	Lack or loss of appetite for food.
contamination:	A state of being made impure by coming into contact with dirty substances, persons or surfaces.
guarding:	This is the tensing of the abdominal wall muscles to protect inflamed organs within the abdomen from the pain of pressure upon them.
lumen:	The hollow inside of the intestines.
nausea:	A feeling of biliousness. A pronounced stomach discomfort and the sensation of wanting to vomit.
tenderness:	Sensitivity to pain that is elicited on pressure.
ulceration:	Formation of a sore on the skin or a mucous membrane, accompanied by the disintegration of tissue.

PREREQUISITE KNOWLEDGE
- Human anatomy and physiology of the gastrointestinal tract.

MEDICO-LEGAL CONSIDERATIONS

Appendicitis is fairly common in children. Appendicitis must be excluded in children presenting with pain that is persistent in the peri-umbilical area. Inappropriate assessment by nurses at the clinic has resulted in late referral, resulting in the appendix having ruptured before it can be operated upon, putting the life of the affected child at risk.

> **ESSENTIAL HEALTH LITERACY**
>
> It is important for families to know about childhood diseases so that they also can be of assistance in seeking medical advice early. Abdominal pain, like upper respiratory tract infection, is a common complaint. Parents must always take time to explore the origins of the pain, when it started, its distribution and nature. A persistent periumbilical pain must always be regarded as serious and must be investigated in the clinic or by a physician.

Introduction

Acute appendicitis is the infection and inflammation of the appendix caused by hardened faecal material that causes obstruction of the lumen of the appendix. The obstruction can also be caused by swollen lymphoid tissue, foreign bodies like threadworms (*Enterobius vermicularis*), tumours of the caecum or adhesions.

Pathophysiology

Once there is an obstruction by faecal matter, lymphoid tissue or threadworms, pressure that builds within the appendix lumen compresses the blood vessels, resulting in poor blood supply to the area. This is followed by ulceration and bacterial infection of the epithelial lining of the lumen. Subsequent necrosis causes perforation with faecal and bacterial contamination of the peritoneal cavity. Progressive inflammation causes obstruction of the ileus, while fluid drawn to the peritoneal cavity as a response to inflammation causes major electrolyte imbalance and hypovoleamic shock.

Clinical manifestation

- The clinical manifestations are mainly pain and its many descriptions.
  - It is a colicky and crampy referred abdominal pain around the umbilical area.
  - The pain becomes progressively constant, having migrated to the right lower quadrant of the abdomen. It is accompanied by abdominal tenderness and 'guarding'. Guarding is a significant sign in peritonitis.
  - Rebound tenderness is pain that is elicited with deep, firm palpitation and when the pressure is released the pain is also relieved.
  - The child may complain of pain in the right hip and may not be able to walk well because of this pain.
- There is also nausea, vomiting and anorexia.
- Diarrhoea may be followed by constipation.
- Poor feeding, lethargy, irritability.
- There might be fever that is not very high, but temperature can increase to 39.4 °C after perforation.

Assessment and common findings

Subjective data consists of the history and physical examination for pain. Other relevant information relates to fever, nausea, anorexia and vomiting.

Objective data consists of a physical examination to locate the pain and link the findings to the subjective description of the pain, such as a raised temperature (39 °C) and a rapid pulse. Laboratory test must include full blood cell count. A white cell count greater than 10,000/mm^3 and an elevated C-reactive protein are common findings characteristic of an infection. Urinalysis to rule out urinary tract infection is also done. Radiographic studies will show a dilated loop of bowel indicative of paralytic ileus, air and fluid levels in case of obstruction and free air in the peritoneum consistent with perforation.

Management of appendicitis

Because of the many signs and symptoms that present with appendicitis, it usually takes time to make a definite diagnosis. A child who is incapacitated by pain around the umbilicus with pain radiating to the lower right quadrant must be investigated for appendicitis. The inflamed appendix may be removed. Appendicectomy may be done through laparotomy or laparoscopy. If an abscess has formed, an incision and drainage may be necessary.

Specific preoperative care

Once the diagnosis has been confirmed:
- administer prescribed analgesics and antibiotics for pain and infection, respectively, in preparation for surgery
- monitor and record vital signs to detect infection early, and response to medication
- withhold oral feeds and, if paralytic ileus or peritonitis has developed, insert a nasogastric tube to drain gastric contents continuously while awaiting surgery
- in preparation for surgery, monitor intravenous therapy to ensure good hydration and a balance of electrolytes because the patient might be vomiting
- explain the activities to the patient and parents/guardians to alleviate anxiety
- obtain consent from parents/guardians after explaining the planned management (appendicectomy).

For perioperative care, see Chapters 3, 4, and 5.

Specific postoperative care

Postoperative care is the same as for all other abdominal procedures:
- Pain management is essential in the care of the child. Prescribed analgesics are administered to ensure that the child does not experience any pain.
- The child is allowed nothing orally until bowel sounds are heard and use of the nasogastric tube is discontinued.
- Intravenous therapy is monitored and maintained as prescribed.
- Antibiotics are administered as prescribed.
- Wound dressing is observed for haemorrhage and the wound drain, if in place, is left until there is no more drainage.
- Vital signs are monitored every 30 minutes in the first 6 hours postoperatively and then 4-hourly to detect any infection early.
- All drainage, output and fluid intake through IV therapy is measured and recorded.
- The wound is aseptically cleaned to minimise the risk of infection.

If there were no complications, such as perforation and peritonitis, recovery postoperatively is within 5 to 7 days.

Potential complications of appendicitis that might impact negatively on the surgery (appendicectomy)

Haemorrhage is a potential complication in all surgical procedures. It may also be indicative of secondary infection. It can have negative outcomes on the child's recovery and parents'/guardians' morale. Apart from aseptic technique perioperatively, infection is dependent on preoperative circumstances such as perforations, presence of peritonitis, or paralytic ileus. The presence of any of these predisposes the child to postoperative infection.

The care plan is the same as that for abdominal surgery.

Table 8.1: Postoperative nursing care plan for a child who has undergone appendicectomy

Problem: Pain	
Nursing diagnosis	• Altered comfort due to pain related to surgery performed evidenced by restlessness, crying, pallor, and if old enough verbal expression of pain
Expected outcome	• No pain
Nursing intervention and rationale	• Assess pain adequately to get baseline data against which to measure progress • Administer analgesics as prescribed to relieve pain • Ensure that all lines are not blocked as these may cause pain if not draining or running well, eg drips should not infiltrate, wound drain should flow freely • Prevent hypothermia. Cover the patient lightly to ensure correct and comfortable temperature • Engage the physiotherapist to support the operated site during breathing and coughing exercises • Help the patient to assume a comfortable position without stretching the incision or pressing on it. This may be a semi-Fowler's position to relive tension on the operated site • Monitor and record vital signs to assess the intensity of the pain experienced so that pain management can be improved.
Evaluation	• Child is sleeping peaceful and responding to sedation. No crying and no pain
Problem: Risk of peritonitis	
Nursing diagnosis	• Risk of peritonitis related to the condition (peritonitis occurs as a result of perforation preoperatively)
Expected outcome	• No peritonitis

Nursing intervention and rationale	• Monitor vital signs and take note and report an increase in the breathing and pulse rates and rhythm. • Administer and record analgesics and antibiotics as prescribed • Retain the nasogastric tube and allow it to drain until bowel sounds are heard and there is no vomiting. • Observe and monitor abdominal distension by measuring the abdominal girth daily until satisfied that abdominal distension does not exist • Monitor and record intravenous infusion to prevent dehydration.
Evaluation	• No pain and no abdominal distension

Problem: Hydration and nutrition

Nursing diagnosis	• Fluid volume deficit and altered nutrition related to preoperative care which requires that the child takes nothing orally, and the naso-gastric suctioning pre and post operatively
Expected outcome	• Child to maintain normal hydration and normal nutrition
Nursing intervention and rationale	• Monitor the intravenous line and administer intravenous fluids as prescribed to maintain hydration. Record fluid intake • Ensure that the naso-gastric tube is draining and record the drainage as fluid output. Leave the nasogastric tube in situ until the bowel sounds are heard and the child is stable and there is no vomiting • Start the intake of oral fluids with small sips and amounts of clear water, followed by expressed breast milk or formula feed or soft diet • Increase the feeds gradually to avoid sudden distension of the stomach.
Evaluation	• Child well hydrated, taking feeds and food satisfactorily and gaining weight as expected

Problem: Risk of anxiety

Nursing diagnosis	• For the parent the risk of anxiety is related to knowledge deficit about the surgery and its outcomes
Expected outcome	• No anxiety

Nursing intervention and rationale	• Provide information and explain the pathology of appendicitis, manifestations, possible prognosis and possible modalities of care and treatment (ie, appendicectomy) to parents/guardian • Provide information about available alternatives to treatment • Refer to physiotherapy to assist with the prescribed exercises • Encourage the parents to talk about the child's condition and allow them to ask questions and to verbalise fears and concerns freely. If parents can accept the situation they are more likely to participate in the care much more willing than they otherwise would • Provide counselling for parents/guardian and refer to the psychologist for further professional counselling if this is deemed necessary.
Evaluation	• Parents able to talk about the child's condition freely and participating in the care

Conclusion

The prognosis for appendicectomy, if presenting by itself with no perforation and peritonitis, is good. The child is usually back to their normal activities by the 2nd week. The crucial aspect is to make the diagnosis on time and to refer the patient directly for appropriate management.

Suggested activities for learners

Activity 8.1
1. In the assessment of a child who might be diagnosed as suffering from appendicitis for appendicectomy, what are the characteristic signs you would look out for to make this diagnosis?
2. Create a nursing care plan for a child post-appendicectomy.

References

Hockenberry, MJ, & Wilson, D. 2015. *Wong's nursing care of infants and children*. 10th edition. Elsevier.

Mogotlane, S, Mokoena, J, Chauke, M, Matlakala, M, Young, A, & Randa, B. 2018. *Juta's complete textbook of medical surgical nursing*. 2nd edition. Cape Town: Juta.

Mott, SR, James, SR, & Sperhac, AM. 1990. *Nursing care of children and families*. 2nd edition. New York: Addison-Wesley Nursing.

9 Tonsillitis, tonsillectomy and adenoidectomy

LEARNING OBJECTIVES

At the end of this Chapter, you should be able to:
- describe the causative factors of tonsillitis
- explain the indications for tonsillectomy and adenoidectomy
- describe the nursing management post-tonsillectomy/adenoidectomy
- describe the care of a tracheostomy in a child.

KEY CONCEPTS AND TERMINOLOGY	
dysphagia:	Pain and difficulty with swallowing.
haemorrhage:	Bleeding.
hoarseness:	Loss of voice.
hyperpyrexia:	Extremely high temperature.
pharyngitis:	Infection and inflammation of the pharynx that could be viral or bacterial in origin.
otalgia:	Pain in the ear.
quinsy:	This is an abscess in the tonsillar area (peritonsillar abscess).

PREREQUISITE KNOWLEDGE
- Anatomy and physiology of the pharynx
- Application of universal precautions; microbiology and parasitology

MEDICO-LEGAL CONSIDERATIONS

Tonsillectomy and adenoidectomy are surgical procedures that are usually performed together. Although these are fairly easy and safe surgical procedures, potential complications of bleeding and infection can result in litigations, where healthcare professionals are accused of failure to conduct due care. Hence observation of swallowing while the child is still unconscious and monitoring of vital signs are very important postoperatively.

ESSENTIAL HEALTH LITERACY

Tonsillectomy and adenoidectomy can be performed as day surgery, where the child

> is sent home soon after operation. Should this be the case, parents/guardians must be cautioned to observe for swallowing actions and bleeding through the mouth. Should this happen, they should contact the health facility responsible immediately.

Introduction

Tonsils and adenoids are lymphoid tissue around the nasopharynx and the oropharynx. Their function is to filter and protect the respiratory and gastrointestinal tracts from invading pathogens. Tonsillitis is the infection and inflammation of the tonsillar tissue that occurs with pharyngitis. The causal organisms are streptococcus and haemophilus influenza. Tonsillitis can be acute or chronic and is common in children between the ages of 4 and 14 years. Chronic tonsillitis is when the tonsils are repeatedly enlarged and infected. Management of tonsillitis can be medical or surgical.

Tonsillectomy is the surgical removal of the palatine tonsils, while adenoidectomy is the removal of the adenoids.

Assessment and common findings

Subjective data
- There may be a history of upper respiratory tract infection.
- The patient may report pain in the throat and difficulty with swallowing (dysphagia) and otalgia (earache).
- The adenoids may be enlarged, resulting in difficulty with breathing. The child may breathe through the mouth speak with a nasal sound, and snore.
- The child presents with hyperpyrexia, resulting in febrile seizures.

Objective data
- There is a visible enlargement of the adenoids at the back of the mouth.
- Breathing is noisy and mouth breathing results in the mouth being dry.
- There may be a purulent discharge from the tonsils. A swab specimen from the purulent discharge will help determine the infecting organisms.

Indications for tonsillectomy are:
- a history of recurrent attacks of acute or chronic tonsillitis
- hypertrophied tonsils or adenoids causing airway obstruction
- repeated otitis media due to obstruction of the Eustachian tube
- one attack of peritonsillar abscess (quinsy)
- tonsillitis resulting in febrile seizures.

Preoperative care

Tonsillectomy is contra-indicated in the acute stage of the infection. It is planned for when the child is free from infection. The nurse needs to take a history of bleeding tendencies and upper respiratory tract infection and report these if present.

For pre- and intraoperative care, see Chapters 3, 4 and 5.

Postoperative care following tonsillectomy

Position. In the ward, the child is placed in the recovery position (exaggerated Sims' position) until they are fully awake and are able to cough and swallow normally (see Figure 9.1 (a) and (b)):

- While the child is still unconscious, observe for swallowing, as this is indicative of bleeding in the operated site.
- When awake, provide child with a kidney dish to spit into. Observe the nature of the spit, and note the amount and nature if bloody and profuse. Report abnormal bleeding to the surgeon.
- Inspect the mouth for the presence of fresh blood and report if observed.
- Monitor vital signs every 15 to 30 minutes for the first 12 to 24 hours for early detection of haemorrhage. A fast, thready pulse and low blood pressure are indicative of haemorrhage.
- Pain in the throat and otalgia should be managed by giving prescribed medication.
- Oral feeds should be commenced as soon as recovery from anaesthesia is complete and the child can tolerate feeds. Give cool drinks and a soft, bland diet. Give toasted bread for breakfast the following day.
- Give antiseptic mouth washes every 4 hours for the first 24 hours.

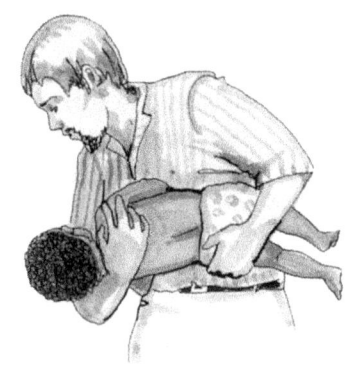

Figure 9.1 (a) Recovery position in an infant

- Keep the airway clear.
- Hand supports head
- Knee stops body from rolling onto the stomach
- Stay with the child. If you must leave them alone at any point, or if they are unconscious, put them in this position to keep airway clear and prevent choking.

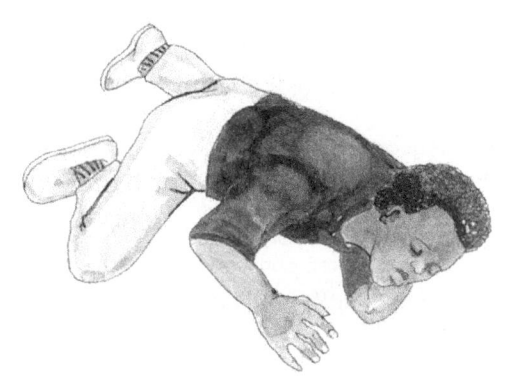

Figure 9.1 (b) Recovery position in an older child

Potential risks post-tonsillectomy:
- **Haemorrhage.** This could occur in the first 12 to 24 hours. The management is to:
  - find the bleeding spot and report to the surgeon as an emergency; child might need to go back to theatre to ligate the bleeding blood vessel
  - get the child to rinse the mouth with an antiseptic mouthwash
  - ensure that the child has assumed the recovery position to avoid aspiration and asphyxiation
  - give antibiotics as prescribed as an infection can also cause haemorrhage.
- **Infection.** This could occur after 24 hours. The management is to:
  - monitor, record and report vital signs, as an increase in these will be an indication of early infection
  - observe for secondary haemorrhage; report as there may be a need to change antibiotics.

Essential patient teaching

Tonsillectomy is a day procedure and, as such, patients are likely to be sent home as soon as they awake from anaesthesia. Therefore, it is important for them to know what needs to be done. Patients are encouraged to see the surgeon if bleeding persists. Patients must also report bleeding occurring after 7 to 10 days, as this is indicative of infection.

Peritonsillar abscess (quinsy)

Peritonsillar abscess occurs with tonsillitis and is a strong indication for tonsillectomy. The presence of peritonsillar abscess is marked by severe pain, a stiff neck, inability to swallow, a hoarse voice and a very high temperature with rigors. The management is surgical incision and drainage, analgesics for pain and broad-spectrum antibiotics. A tonsillectomy is done when the peritonsillar abscess has been resolved.

Table 9.1 Postoperative nursing care plan for tonsillectomy

Problem: Pain	
Nursing diagnosis	• Altered comfort due to pain (sore throat) related to surgery performed evidenced by restlessness, crying, pallor, and if old enough verbal expression of pain on swallowing
Expected outcome	• No sore throat
Nursing intervention and rationale	• Assess pain adequately to get baseline data against which to measure progress • Administer analgesics as prescribed to relieve pain • Prevent hypothermia. Cover the patient lightly to ensure correct and comfortable temperature • Instruct patient to refrain from too much talking as this may cause throat pain.
Evaluation	• No pain. Child able to swallow

Problem: Risk of haemorrhage	
Nursing diagnosis	• Fluid volume deficit due to bleeding related to surgery
Expected outcome	• No bleeding
Nursing intervention and rationale	• Put child in a prone or recovery position with the head turned to the side to allow for drainage of blood from the mouth • While the child is unconscious, observe for the swallowing action. If present report to the surgeon • Monitor vital signs quarter hourly. If pulse thready, and rapid observe for swallowing actions and report on these. If child awake give a basin or tissues to expectorate into and report and record untoward amounts • Prepare for the examination of the surgical site and packing of the wound.
Evaluation	• No bleeding. Vital signs normal
Problem: Risk of infection	
Nursing diagnosis	• Risk of wound infection related to surgery, evidenced by secondary bleeding and a raised temperature, pulse and respiration
Expected outcome	• No bleeding. Vital signs normal
Nursing intervention and rationale	• Monitor vital signs and take note and report increased temperature, pulse and respiration • Administer and record analgesics and antibiotics as prescribed • Rinse mouth with salt water/
Evaluation	• No bleeding. Vital signs normal
Problem: Hydration and nutrition	
Nursing diagnosis	• Fluid volume deficit and altered nutrition related to pain on swallowing
Expected outcome	• Maintain normal hydration and normal nutrition
Nursing intervention and rationale	• Offer cool water to drink and ice tubes to suck if there is no bleeding. Record fluid intake • Start on food intake as soon as desired.
evaluation	• Hydration satisfactory and gaining weight as expected

Care of a child with tracheostomy

Tracheostomy is the surgical creation of a stoma or opening into the trachea (between the third and fourth tracheal rings) to create an artificial airway. It is a form of management of upper airway obstruction and can be performed as an emergency or elective procedure. In chronic tracheostomy, the patient needs to be counselled and supported to take charge of self-management. They are taught and encouraged to suction themselves as well as do the dressings. This is done to allow them a sense of control over themselves and not to be dependent on others. The patient will have difficulty in producing sound, and there is a need to refer them for speech therapy for assistance with sound and speech.

Indications for a tracheostomy

- To relieve acute or chronic upper airway obstruction as a result of:
  - congenital webs or atresia of the trachea
  - laryngeal oedema, laryngeal spasm in acute laryngotracheobronchitis
  - impaction of a foreign body in the larynx
  - chronic stenosis of the larynx following burns
  - bilateral abductor paralysis of the vocal cords following injury to the recurrent laryngeal nerve
- to facilitate access for continuous mechanical ventilation in conditions such as
  - unconsciousness associated with head injury
- to improve respiratory function by enabling effective aspiration of bronchial secretions in conditions such as
  - bronchopneumonia
  - chronic bronchitis
  - chest injuries, particularly flail chest
- to improve respiration in cases where there is respiratory paralysis, such as
  - bulbar-type poliomyelitis
  - unconsciousness
  - tetanus
- to relieve irritation where the tracheal tube has been in place for a long time and has eroded the mucous membrane in the larynx.

Potential problems of a tracheostomy

- **Bleeding and coughing.** The surgeon must put a plan in place to control bleeding. The suctioning should be done gently so that the catheter does not initiate coughing bouts.
- **Crusting in the trachea.** This is cleaned with the aid of a bronchoscope, which is passed through the stoma.
- **Obstruction.** As a result of oedema, tube obstruction or accidental dislodgement of the tube.
- **Surgical emphysema.** This occurs if the tracheostomy tube slips into the tissues of the neck.
- **Pneumothorax.** This is when free air is sucked into the pleural cavity. It is indicated by the presence of dysponea and cyanosis.
- Also see Table 9.2.

Table 9.2 Complications of a tracheostomy

Complication	Recognition	Action	Prevention
Obstruction	• Stridor • Intercostal recession • Tracheal tug	• Add or increase oxygen • Call for assistance • Deflate cuff • Pass suction catheter • Remove inner tube • Nebulise the patient with saline	• Humidification • Regular suctioning • Cleaning the inner tube • Maintaining patient hydration • Checking cuff pressure
Displacement	• Surgical emphysema • Altered tube position • Signs of obstruction	• Give oxygen if tube is out • Keep dilators next to the patient at all times • Keep stoma open with tracheal dilators	• Check tapes at start of each shift • Change tapes daily • Observe central tube position
Haemorrhage	• Bleeding from stoma site • Clots on suction • Copious blood on suction • Respiratory distress	• Increase oxygen • Inflate cuff, if present • Attempt suctioning • Consider tilting head down	• Ensure that the tube is centrally situated • Ensure tube is secure • Avoid trauma during tracheal care and suctioning

Principles of tracheostomy care
- Maintaining patient safety
- Facilitating communication
- Prevention of complications

The main purpose of a tracheostomy is to ensure free air entry. The site should therefore be suctioned regularly to achieve this purpose. It should be cleaned regularly with saline solution and dressed with dry gauze dressings, which should be changed whenever soiled. Periodic humidification is essential to keep the airway moist and prevent crust formation.

> **Clinical alert!**
> The tracheostomy tube is securely held in place by tape that is changed whenever soiled or worn out.

Conclusion
Patients with a chronic tracheostomy need to be counselled and supported to take charge of themselves. They are taught and encouraged to suction themselves as well as do their own dressings. This allows them to develop a sense of control over themselves and not to

be dependent on others. Patients also find it difficult to produce sound, so there is a need to refer them for speech therapy for assistance with sound production and speech.

> **Suggested activities for learners**
>
> **Activity 9.1**
> 1. Outline the indications for tonsillectomy.
> 2. Explain why and how you would suspect bleeding in a child post-tonsillectomy.
> 3. What are the recommended positions to assume post-tonsillectomy and why?
> 4. Outline the potential problems in tracheostomy and how any two of these are managed.

References

Hockenberry, MJ, & Wilson, D. 2015. *Wong's nursing care of infants and children*. 10th edition. Elsevier.

Mogotlane, S, Mokoena, J, Chauke, M, Matlakala, M, Young, A, & Randa, B. 2018. *Juta's complete textbook of medical surgical nursing*. 2nd edition. Cape Town: Juta.

Mott, SR, James, SR, & Sperhac, AM. 1990. *Nursing care of children and families*. 2nd edition. New York: Addison-Wesley Nursing.

10 The child and trauma: fractures

LEARNING OBJECTIVES

At the end of this Chapter, you should be able to:
- explain the various types of fractures, their causes, signs and symptoms and management
- make accurate assessment in patients with fractures
- manage emergencies and complications resulting from fractures.

KEY CONCEPTS AND TERMINOLOGY	
amputation:	Severing of a limb or finger/toe.
callus:	A hard tissue that forms around the edges of broken bone.
contractures:	Abnormal tightening or shortening of muscles, tendons or ligaments across a joint, inhibiting movement in the affected joint. Muscles may also tighten around the intestines following abdominal surgery, forming bands that may cause obstruction.
diaphysis:	This is the shaft or centre part of a long bone.
epiphysis:	The end part of a long bone.
fracture:	A break or bend in the continuity of a bone.
metaphysis:	That part of the long bone between the epiphysis and the diaphysis.
ossification:	A process of bone hardening.
periosteum:	Thick bone covering with osteoblasts on inner surface (bone facing side) and blood vessels on the outer surface.
phantom limb:	This is a sensation that an amputated limb is still in place and the person feels pain.
osteoblasts:	Bone-forming cells found on the inner surface of the periosteum.
prosthesis:	An artificial body part structured to resemble the original part.
splint:	A support mechanism.

stump:	On the human body, this serves to describe a part of the body that is left behind following an amputation or, in congenital defects, this is a blind end in tubular structures.

PREREQUISITE KNOWLEDGE
- Human anatomy and physiology of the musculoskeletal system
- Biophysics

MEDICO-LEGAL CONSIDERATIONS

Trauma in children is commonly caused by lack of judgement and inexperience. This may cause debility, which in some cases may result in permanent deformities. In hospital, it is important that children are nursed in closed cot beds to prevent falls from rolling or jumping over the edge. The environment where children are and the play which they engage in must be supervised at all times and the flooring must be non-slip. Any injury sustained during hospitalisation becomes the hospital's responsibility and needs to be investigated.

Introduction

Bone injury can be a result of accidental falls or twists, most of which occur during general play or organised play, or from more traumatic causes like motor vehicle accidents. Bone injury as a result of a blow should be investigated to exclude child abuse. Bones prone to fractures are the clavicle, humerus, radius, ulna and femur. In neonates, fractures of the clavicle may occur during birth if the baby is large and delivery has to be manipulated. Table 10.1 provides a classification of fractures.

Table 10.1 Classification of fractures

Type of fracture	Description of the fracture
Complete fracture	This is when the bone fragments are separated into two or more parts. This type can be closed or open, depending on the status of the muscles and skin around the fracture
Incomplete fracture	When the fragments remain attached but the bone bends over, eg greenstick fracture (see Figure 10.1)
Described in lines	This is when a fracture occurs along a line. The line may describe the nature of the fracture, which it can be complete or incomplete
• transverse	• Crosswise at right angles to the long axis of the bone
• oblique	• Slanting but straight
• spiral	• Circular and twisting around the bone.

Skin status	This describes whether the fracture does or does not involve the skin and tissues around it
• simple/closed	• This is a fracture with no break in the skin. The fracture may be complete or incomplete
• compound/open complicated	• These are fractures where there is a wound and the bone protrudes through
• comminuted	• This is a fracture where the bone fragments cause damage to tissues. The fragments of bone may be lodged in the surrounding tissues.

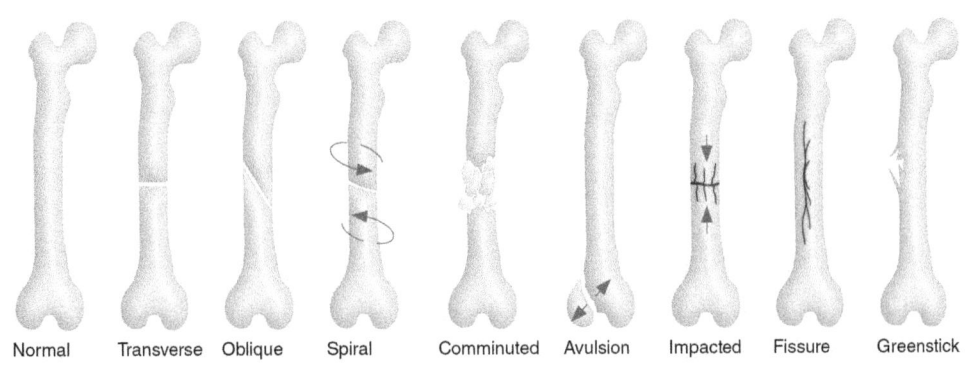

Figure 10.1 Types of fracture in children

Clinical manifestations of a fracture
Cardinal signs of a fracture include pain, swelling at the site of the fracture, shortening of the limb and loss of function. A child will not move a fractured part. If the injury is to the lower limbs in walking children, they will not walk. In crawling infants, any fracture of the clavicle will mean the child will not crawl.

Bone healing in children
Bone healing in children occurs fairly quickly because of the thick periosteum and good blood supply. When a bone breaks, the periosteal and intraosseous osteoblasts are stimulated to produce new osteoblasts immediately between the bone fragments. This is followed by deposition of calcium salts to form callus. The typical time it takes for callus to form in the femur at different ages in childhood are as follows:
- neonatal period: 2–3 weeks
- early childhood: 4 weeks
- late childhood: 6–8 weeks
- adolescence: 8–12 weeks.

Table 10.2 Types of fracture

Type of fracture	Explanation
Plastic deformation	In this type of fracture the bone is bent.
Buckle fracture	This is a fracture that occurs at the porous portion of the bone near the metaphysis.
Greenstick fracture	This is when the bone is bent to the extent that it becomes an incomplete fracture.
Complete fracture	The bone fragments divide into two but remain attached by the periosteum.

Management of a fracture

The aim of the management of a fracture is to align the fractured fragments, immobilise these and maintain the immobility. This will assist in controlling pain and facilitate union.

First aid:
- Use appropriate splinting devices to minimise movement and relieve pain. The splints range from a simple back slab to those used for skeletal traction. To promote comfort, the splint is padded and a bandage may be applied lightly to stabilise the body part. Other immobilising devices include braces that are worn to support the body and to prevent further injury.

Further management:
- Administer prescribed analgesics to control pain.
- Replace fluid: depending on the type and extent of the fracture, there might be bleeding and shock:

- Maintain intravenous infusion.
- Monitor vital signs to assess blood loss, low blood pressure and a thready pulse, as they are indicative of pending shock. To manage this, blood and blood products are administered, depending on the haemoglobin level.

> **Box 10.1 Stages of bone healing**
>
> **Stage 1 – haematoma formation.** When a break in the bone occurs, surrounding tissues, muscle and periosteum are torn, blood vessels rupture, bleeding into tissues occurs and a haematoma forms even around the bone fragments.
> **Stage 2 – cellular proliferation.** Blood supply increases, bringing calcium, phosphate and fibroblasts. Cells proliferate at the ends of bone fragments and differentiate into cartilage and connective tissue. In a few days the fibroblasts convert to osteoblasts. This takes 2 to 3 days.
> **Stage 3 – callus formation.** Within about 6 to 10 days, calcium and phosphorus are deposited onto the osteoblasts and callus develops. Callus resembles bone tissue, but will not support body weight. It is opaque and pliable.
> **Stage 4 – ossification.** Within about 3 to 10 weeks, callus forms into bone, which grows from underneath the periosteum.
> **Stage 5 – consolidation and remodelling.** By the 9th month, compact bone forms and remodelling occurs.

Reduction of the fracture
Reduction of the fracture occurs when the displaced bone ends are brought into alignment.

Specific preoperative care
Care is the same as the general perioperative care discussed in Chapters 3, 4 and 5.

Some orthopaedic specialists may require the skin to be prepared, in which case they usually state how this is to be done. In some instances, the fractured bone is immobilised and no open surgery is done, eg a fractured clavicle is treated by putting the arm and hand in a shoulder sling for a month, periodically taking the arm out of the sling to do passive joint movements to prevent contractures.

Closed reduction
This is the manual realignment of the fractured bones, or the process putting a piece of a broken bone back together in the right position. It can be done under local or general anaesthesia, after which the limb is immobilised using a cast, traction, splint or bandages to maintain the alignment. An X-ray of the affected part is taken and the immobilisation effected as prescribed.

Open reduction
This is usually done under anaesthesia. The fracture fragments are exposed surgically by dissecting the tissues, and the fractured bone fragments are aligned using screws, nails, pins and wires. It is often called open reduction and internal fixation (ORIF).

Types of casts

Open cast. This is a slab-like device made of plaster of Paris (POP), or the slab is a cylinder-like device cut into half lengthwise.

Closed cast. This cast is usually prepared for the limbs and includes the upper or lower part of the body. It is closed and cylindrical and wraps around a limb.

Short arm cast. This cast extends from below the elbow to the palmar crease and may be secured around the thumb. It is used to immobilise fractures of the arm, wrist and hand (see Figure 10.2).

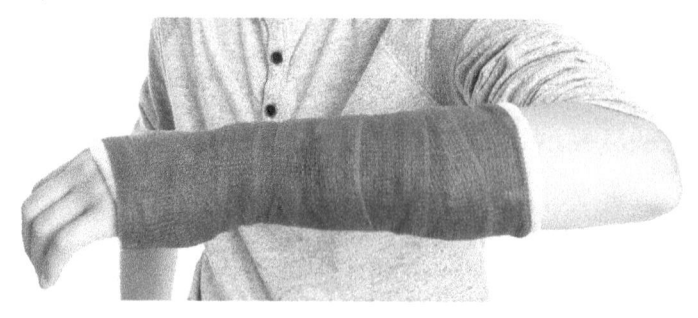

Figure 10.2 Short arm cast

Thumb spica. This cast is used to support a fractured thumb (see Figure 10.3).

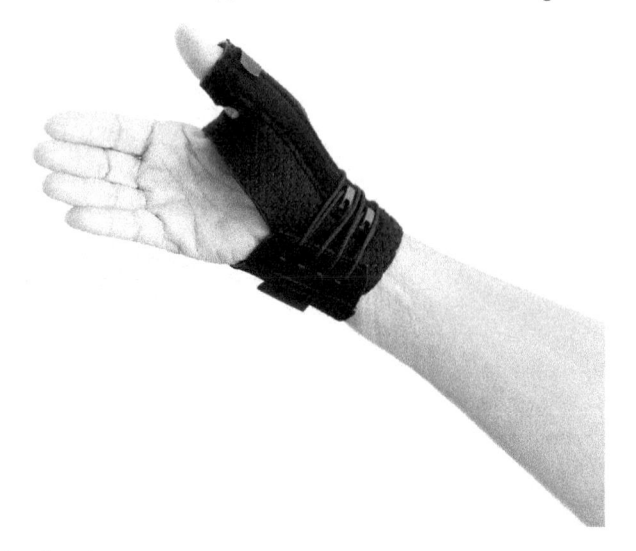

Figure 10.3 Thumb spica

Long arm cast. This cast extends over the whole length of the arm. The elbow is immobilised at an angle (see Figure 10.4).

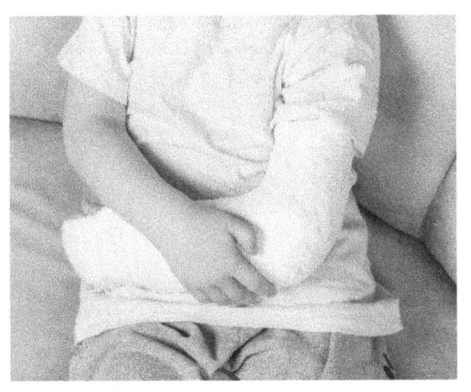

Figure 10.4 Long arm cast

Shoulder spica. This cast encloses the upper trunk, shoulder and elbow (see Figure 10.5).

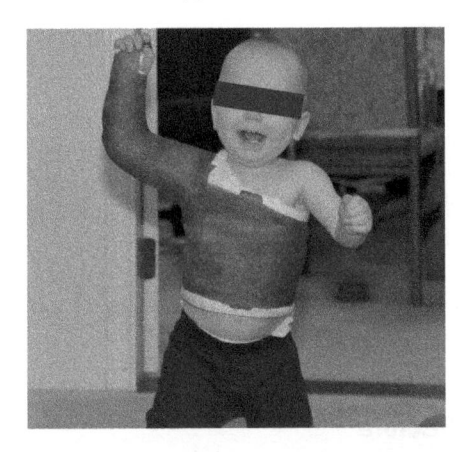

Figure 10.5 Shoulder spica

Long leg cast. This cast extends over the whole length of the leg (see Figure 10.6).

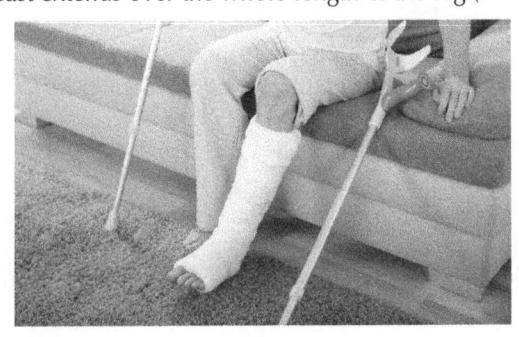

Figure 10.6 Long leg cast

Hip spica: This cast encloses the lower trunk and the lower extremity or extremities (see Figure 10.7).

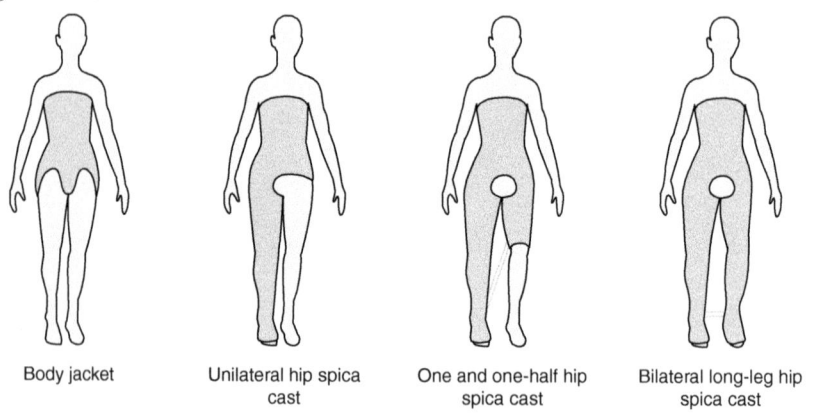

Body jacket | Unilateral hip spica cast | One and one-half hip spica cast | Bilateral long-leg hip spica cast

Figure 10.7 Hip spica

Postoperative care

The aim is to immobilise the fracture to maintain the aligned position of the bone ends until union and/or healing takes place. This is done by:
- restricting movement through the use of splints, traction and bandages – a physiotherapist may be enlisted to help the child move under supervision
- supervised mobility, for example, with the use of crutches
- controlling pain by giving analgesics
- monitoring vital signs to diagnose infection early
- observing circulation beyond the reduced area.

> **Practice alert!**
> With modern advances, internal fixation in long bone fractures is the management of choice. Pins and/or plates are placed in the shaft of the long bone to stabilise the body weight, allowing the bone to heal.

Complications of a fracture

- **Infection.** This is common in compound fractures, where the tissues around the fracture have been damaged and there is an open wound. The infection may spread to underlying bony structures, causing osteomyelitis.
- **Delayed union.** This is where the union of the fractured fragments is delayed. This may be due to poor blood supply or inadequate mobilisation/physiotherapy.
- **Malunion.** This is when the fragments are not properly aligned during the reduction or as a result of contractures that form.
- **Non-union.** This is when the fracture fails to resolve as a result of poor blood supply or inadequate mobilisation.
- **Persistent pain.** This may indicate any of the complications already outlined above.
- **Contractures.** This is an abnormal shortening of muscle, tendon or ligament due to lack of exercise during the period a fracture is immobilised or malalignment when the fracture is set.

Amputation

Amputation refers to the severing of limbs, fingers and toes. Children may be born with congenital absence of body parts such as an arm or foot, experience a traumatic loss of an extremity or extremities in motor vehicle accidents, or require a surgical amputation for a pathological condition such as osteosarcoma. Amputation can be an emergency or an elective surgical procedure. Congenital absence of body parts is not considered as amputation, and those affected have to be treated differently from those requiring surgery to remove body parts.

In amputations, the surgeon aims at constructing an adequately nourished residual limb with a stump that is smooth and well padded, with no nerve endings that would impede prosthesis fitting.

For preoperative care, refer to Chapters 3, 4 and 5.

Specific preoperative care

If the child is old enough, preoperative care mainly involves counselling and support by professionals such as psychologists, occupational therapists and social workers to prepare the child for life without a body part. The child and their parents/guardians need to understand how the patient's body image will have changed postoperatively. They need to know about the 'phantom limb' phenomenon, so that they are not surprised by this experience. It is important to let them know that prostheses can be fitted to the stump to make up for the missing part and that the child will be trained to adapt to the prosthesis. The child and family need to choose the prosthesis and be satisfied with its texture and colour. The counsellor may introduce the child and family to other amputees for group support.

Specific postoperative care

Postoperative care in the case of a lower limb amputations is as follows (also see Table 10.3):

- The stump must be cleaned and dressed aseptically until healed. An elastic bandage applied in a figure of eight in a conical fashion is used to apply compression to the new stump to control haemorrhage, reduce oedema and assist in the development of desired contours to shape the stump for further management. The stump may be elevated for 24 hours to assist in the reduction of oedema. Once the oedema is reduced, the stump can be supported on a pillow.
- The child is nursed in a cot bed to avoid falls, especially when they experience the phantom limb phenomenon. The phantom pain must be treated appropriately with analgesics, because this is real pain in the mind of the amputee.
- Monitor body alignment to prevent contractures. Turn the child to lie in a prone or recumbent position.
- For mobilisation, the joint above the amputation must be moved through a full range of motion no less than twice daily; a monkey chain must be fitted on the frame of the bed to allow an older child to facilitate mobility and prevent pressure sores. A young child is spontaneously active and must be encouraged to move.
- A prosthesis must be fitted as soon as possible, and the child is to be encouraged to walk on the prosthesis. Persistent pain could be due to an ill-fitting prosthesis, weakness or joint instability, injury to nerve endings at the stump, or fibrosis of soft tissues. Observations to be made include skin irritation and infection at the stump.

Potential problems:
- The immediate problem after amputation is haemorrhage
- A subsequent potential problem is infection
- Depression about disfigurement may occur.

Table 10.3 Nursing care plan for a child who has had a fractured limb reduced

Problem: Pain	
Nursing diagnosis	• Altered comfort and activity intolerance related to the fracture, pain from soft tissue damage and surgery performed evidenced by restlessness, crying and, if old enough, verbal expression of pain by the patient
Expected outcome	• Patient restful, no crying, and, if old enough, verbalising comfort and no pain • The limb is correctly aligned.
Nursing intervention and rationale	• Assess pain adequately to get baseline data against which to measure progress • Administer analgesics as prescribed to relieve pain • Immobilise limb correctly and maintain alignment. • If the limb is in traction, ensure that correct weights are used, that the limb is suspended correctly and the child's body is correctly aligned • Engage the physiotherapist to help with supervised mobility • Monitor and record vital signs to identify the intensity of pain and other related factors such as haemorrhage and infection, which could be the cause of pain and discomfort.
Evaluation	• Child is sleeping peaceful and responding to sedation. The child is not crying
Problem: Swelling	
Nursing diagnosis	• Altered comfort and risk of altered tissue perfusion related to the inflammatory response following reduction evidenced by the swelling at the point of reduction and expression of pain
Expected outcome	• Swelling subsides
Nursing intervention and rationale	• If possible, the limb is elevated on pillows to improve venous return and reduce swelling • Apply bandages, splints and traction to further provide support to reduce swelling.
Evaluation	• Swelling is subsiding

Problem: Haemorrhage	
Nursing diagnosis	• Fluid volume deficit due to bleeding evidenced by blood-stained dressings, tachycardia, low blood pressure and increased respiratory rate
Expected outcome	• No bleeding
Nursing intervention and rationale	• Monitor vital signs half-hourly for 6 hours post-reduction and, if stable, this can be done every 4 hours. Should the pulse become rapid and weak, report to the surgeon, as this could be an indication of bleeding as a result of poor ligation of blood vessels or secondary infection
• Observe the dressing for any bleeding. If the dressing is soaked with blood add other dressing to serve as pressure on the bleeding surface and report to the surgeon
• Ensure that the intravenous infusion and/or transfusion are administered as prescribed and keep a record of the intake and output to monitor hydration.
Evaluation	• Normal vital signs
• No bleeding observed.
Problem: Immobility	
Nursing diagnosis	• Impaired mobility related to the fracture
Expected outcome	• Range of movement of affected joints restored and maintained
• Range of movement of unaffected joints maintained
• No contractures at joints observed.
Nursing intervention and rationale	• Encourage active movement of joints to prevent contractures and assess joints for stiffness and muscles for weakness
• Engage the services of a physiotherapist for passive movement of joints
• Change position as often as is necessary to prevent pressure sores.
Evaluation	• Patient able to do exercises and regaining mobility
Problem: Risk of infection	
Nursing diagnosis	• Risk of wound infection related to reduction and immobility
Expected outcome	• No signs of infection

Nursing intervention and rationale	• Monitor vital signs and take note and report increased temperature, breathing rate and rhythm • Administer and record analgesics and antibiotics as prescribed • Maintain asepsis when attending to the wound and report any bleeding, pain and inflammation • Apply dressing to support the wound • Monitor and record intravenous infusions to prevent dehydration • Ensure adequate nutrition to build up immunity and support tissue growth and thus wound healing.
Evaluation	• No evidence of infection • Normal vital signs.

Problem: Nutrition

Nursing diagnosis	• Fluid volume deficit and altered nutrition related to pain and general malaise and anxiety about the outcome
Expected outcome	• Maintain normal hydration and normal nutrition
Nursing intervention and rationale	• Monitor the intravenous line and administer intravenous fluids as prescribed to maintain hydration. Record fluid intake • Start the intake of oral feeds soon, ie breast milk or formula feed as well as solid general ward food to maintain the child's nutritional status • Monitor the child's weight as an indicator for good nutrition.
Evaluation	• Child well-hydrated and gaining weight as expected

Problem: Risk of anxiety

Nursing diagnosis	• For the parent/guardian, the risk of anxiety is related to knowledge deficit about the prognosis of the fracture
Expected outcome	• No anxiety
Nursing intervention and rationale	• Provide information and explain the prognosis in fractures, the modalities of care and the treatment to parents/guardians. In a small child, show pictures of the fracture and invite children who have had a fracture and are still in the ward for the child and parents to see and hear from them how they coped and that a fracture does heal

	• Refer to physiotherapy for assistance with the prescribed exercises • Encourage the parents/guardians to talk about the child's condition and allow them to ask questions and to verbalise fears and concerns freely. If parents/guardians can accept the situation they are more likely to participate in the care much more willingly than they otherwise would • Provide counselling for parents/guardians and refer to the psychologist for further professional counselling if this is deemed necessary.
Evaluation	• Parents/guardians are able to talk about the child's condition freely and participate in the care
Problem: Disfigurement	
Nursing diagnosis	• Risk of altered body image secondary to trauma, surgery, scars, contractures, poor posture or poor gait • Anxiety related to injury.
Expected outcome	• Child and parents/guardians have accepted the changes in appearance without anxiety • Child and parents/guardians are participating in the rehabilitation plan.
Nursing intervention and rationale	• Encourage the child and parents/guardians to express feelings about changes in appearance, role and lifestyle and the rehabilitation plan. • Clarify misconceptions about limitations of mobility and activity, and provide information about assistive devices, their use, durability and maintenance • Encourage exercises for both the child and parents/guardians and refer accordingly, such as to the physiotherapist for pain and contracture management; the plastic surgeon for reconstruction surgery if necessary; the psychologist for counselling on how to cope with the injury and its management.
Evaluation	• Child and parents/guardians are participating in the rehabilitation plan and talking freely about the child's circumstances and appearance

Conclusion

Children are vulnerable when it comes to trauma. Because of their lack of experience of trauma and their curiosity, they need constant supervision, even in play. This means guardians and carers have to be vigilant when taking care of children to avoid preventable injuries such as fractures from falls.

Suggested activities for learners

Activity 10.1
Please indicate if the following sentences are **true** or **false**.
Instruction: Rewrite the sentences on a separate sheet of paper. Next to each sentence write either 'true' or 'false'.
1. The following show the period it takes for callus formation in the femur at different ages in childhood:
   (a) Neonatal period: 2–3 weeks
   (b) Early childhood: 4 weeks
   (c) Late childhood: 4–5 weeks
   (d) Adolescence 8–12 weeks
2. (a) Amputation relates to the cutting away of a body part.
   (b) Potential problems in amputations are haemorrhage, infection and disfigurement.
   (c) A splint is used to provide internal fixation of a fracture.
   (d) The child should be encouraged to walk on the prosthesis immediately once it is fitted.
3. The following is true of a fracture EXCEPT:
   Instruction: Rewrite only the incorrect sentences on a separate sheet of paper.
   (a) A greenstick fracture is when the bone is bent to the extent that it becomes an incomplete fracture.
   (b) In a complete fracture the bone fragments divide into two but remain attached by the periosteum.
   (c) A compound fracture is when there are circular and twisting lines indicating cracks around the bone.
   (d) A simple fracture is when there is a complete or incomplete fracture but no break in the skin.
   (e) A complete fracture is when the bone fragments are separated into two or more parts.

References

Hockenberry, MJ, & Wilson, D. 2015. *Wong's nursing care of infants and children*. 10th edition. Elsevier.

Mogotlane, S, Mokoena, J, Chauke, M, Matlakala, M, Young, A, & Randa, B. 2018. *Juta's complete textbook of medical surgical nursing*. 2nd edition. Cape Town: Juta.

Mott, SR, James, SR, & Sperhac AM. 1990. *Nursing care of children and families*. 2nd edition. New York: Addison-Wesley Nursing.

11 Surgical conditions of the central nervous system: hydrocephalus

LEARNING OBJECTIVES

On completion of this Chapter, you should be able to:
- describe the pathophysiology, causes and clinical manifestations of hydrocephalus
- describe the assessment and common findings in patients presenting with hydrocephalus
- accurately interpret assessment findings from diagnostic tests and procedures
- effectively plan, implement and evaluate nursing care, based on assessment and common findings for patients with hydrocephalus.

KEY CONCEPTS AND TERMINOLOGY

ataxia:	Difficulty and poor coordination in walking.
consciousness:	Ability to perceive, interpret and react to stimuli.
hydrocephalus:	Accumulation of fluid in the form of cerebrospinal fluid in the ventricles of the brain.
intracranial pressure:	A measure of the brain tissue and the cerebrospinal fluid that cushions and surrounds the brain.
opisthotonus:	A state of severe hyperextension and spasticity of the back muscles, causing backward arching of the head, back and spine.
reflex:	An action that is performed as a response to stimulus and without conscious thought.

PREREQUISITE KNOWLEDGE

- Anatomy and physiology of the central nervous system
- Applied psychology

MEDICO-LEGAL CONSIDERATIONS

Child safety should always be a priority in planned nursing care. Patients, especially children, with conditions that impact on their level of consciousness and have a potential to be restless must always be cared for in a cot bed to avoid falls.

> **ESSENTIAL HEALTH LITERACY**
> Children diagnosed with hydrocephalus have many health needs. It is helpful for parents/guardians to participate fully in their care while in hospital so that they can learn under supervision. First, parents/guardians have to understand the anatomy and physiology of hydrocephalus and that almost all systems are affected by the condition. The observations that they have to make and the outcomes they have to interpret at home are critical for the child's survival. These include persistent vomiting, poor feeding, elevated temperature, decreased responsiveness and seizures.

Introduction

Hydrocephalus is the enlargement of the head due to an abnormal accumulation of the cerebrospinal fluid (CSF) within the ventricles of the brain.

Pathophysiology. The cerebrospinal fluid is secreted by the choroid plexus into the lateral ventricles of the brain. It then passes through the foramina of Monro into the third ventricle. From there, it flows through the aqueduct of Sylvius into the fourth ventricle. From the fourth ventricle the CSF drains into the lateral foramina of Luschka and midline foramina of Magendie into the cisterna magna. From there, it is distributed into the cerebral and cerebellar subarachnoid spaces, where it is absorbed. This is the circulation of the CSF within the ventricles of the brain (see Figure 11.1).

Hydrocephalus is caused by increased production of CSF that does not balance absorption, impaired absorption of the CSF or obstruction in its circulatory system. These impediments may be congenital where there are malformations in the foramena such as atresia or stenosis, or acquired factors where obstruction follows infections (which when they heal form scars) or tumours. The ventricles dilate and in children the intracranial pressure increases, the skull bone becomes thin, and the cranial suture line widens, resulting in a big head. If this happens after the suture line is set in an older child, the intracranial pressure increases together with other neurologic signs.

Types of hydrocephalus

These can be communicating/non-obstructive and non-communicating/obstructive, depending on the pathology. It can also be classified as congenital or acquired.

Clinical manifestations. In infancy, the head grows at an abnormally fast rate and its measurement may cross one or more percentile lines to reach up to the 95th percentile on the Road to Health Chart, fontanelles are bulging, the skull becomes thin, scalp veins are dilated and standing out, the suture line is palpable, there is frontal bossing with depressed eyes, which may be rotated downwards, producing a 'setting-sun sign' with the sclera visible above the iris (see Figure 11.2). Pupils are sluggish and respond unequally to light. The infant is irritable and lethargic, feeds poorly and therefore does not thrive, and may display changes in the level of consciousness. In extreme cases there may be opisthotonus and lower limb spasticity. Infantile reflexes may persist.

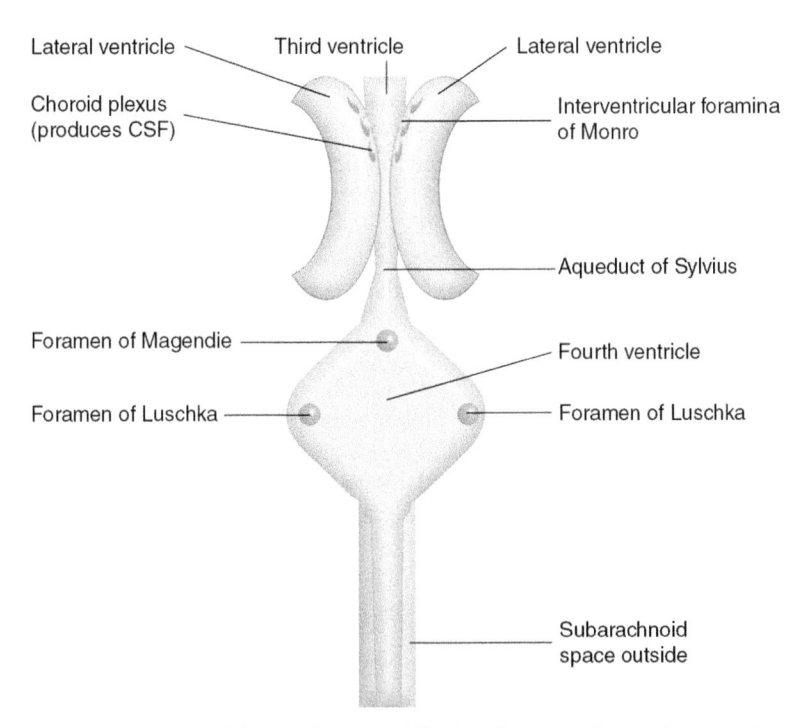

Chapter 11 – Surgical conditions of the central nervous system: hydrocephalus 145

Figure 11.1 Circulation of the cerebrospinal fluid in the ventricles and brain substance

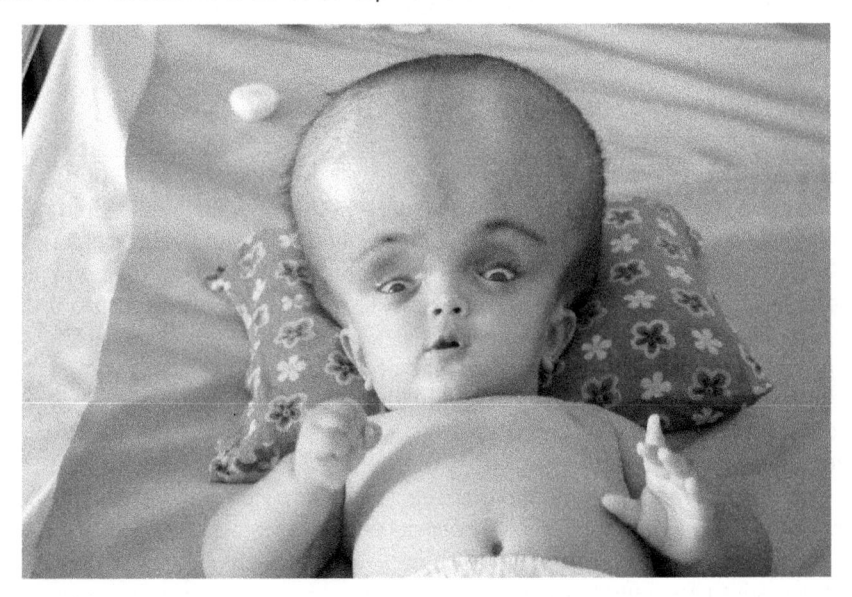

Figure 11.2 Hydrocephalus with the setting-sun sign

In childhood, the signs and symptoms are caused by an increase in intracranial pressure. The child may complain of a headache on waking, the headache is relieved by vomiting, and the child is irritable, lethargic, ataxic, confused and incoherent.

The accumulation of CSF may also compress the brainstem. The child may display behaviour that shows cranial nerve dysfunction, such as arm weakness, dysphagia, stridor and apnoea. Other signs that depict progression include poor feeding, failure to thrive, a high-pitched shrill cry, vomiting and seizures.

In preterm infants, there may be no clinical signs other than the gradual increase in the head circumference. A CT scan and an MRI will be done to confirm the diagnosis, localise the defect and outline the size.

Management
Aim of treatment is to relieve ventricular pressure and treat associated complications.

Obstruction is removed surgically, and in case of overproduction, a mechanism is provided to drain the CSF from the ventricles to an extracranial location, usually the peritoneum. To achieve this, a radio-opaque ventriculoperitoneal shunt, which is easily traceable, is put in place.

11.1 The shunt system

The system consists of a ventricular catheter with a flush pump, a one-way flow valve and a distal catheter. A reservoir may be added to allow for the administration of medication. The valve is set to open at different intraventricular pressures to allow for automatic excess CSF drainage. There are two types of shunts, namely:
- ventriculoperitoneal shunt: from the lateral ventricle into the peritoneum
- ventriculoatrial shunt: from the lateral ventricle to the atrium of the heart.

Specific preoperative care
Surgery can be planned, or this could be an emergency, depending on the circumstances. The child is observed for increasing ventricular size and increasing intercranial pressure:
- The head is measured daily at the largest fronto-occipital diameter. The point at which the tape is wrapped is marked with a marker around the head to ensure that the circumference is measured consistently
- Fontanelles are palpated daily for size and fullness
- Suture lines are palpated to detect splitting or separation, which is an indication of progression of pathology
- Vital signs are monitored
- Hydration and feeding are monitored because there may be failure to thrive
- Observe for changes in the levels of consciousness.

For perioperative care, refer to Chapters 3, 4 and 5.

Specific post-operative care

In addition to routine postoperative care and observation:
- The child is positioned flat on the unoperated side to prevent pressure on the shunt valve. The flat position will prevent the pressure from dropping rapidly after shunting. Pillows are used to maintain the position so that the child does not roll over
- Observe for signs of increased intracranial pressure, such as restlessness, drowsiness and a headache in an older child
- Measure the head circumference daily
- Monitor vital signs to detect infection early
- Observe for abdominal distention, which could be an indication of displacement, or the draining CSF may cause peritonitis or paralytic ileus
- A child that has a ventriculoperitoneal shunt is kept nil per os until bowel sounds are heard
- Monitor fluid and electrolyte balance by measuring and recording the intake and output, recording the specific gravity of urine and maintaining the rate of flow for the intravenous infusion to prevent fluid overload.

> **Clinical alert!**
>
> One of the most devastating postoperative complications is infection. The nurse needs to be on the alert for this and report high temperatures (39 °C), poor feeding, vomiting, decreased responsiveness and seizures.

Complications of shunts

- Shunts are prone to complications such as kinking, blocking by particulate matter, separation and tube migration.
- The main problems based on this are:
  - infection, including wound sepsis, meningitis and brain abscess
  - malfunction when there is obstruction, or displacement.

Discharge plan

Family health education

Children with hydrocephalus have many health needs. The aim is to establish realistic goals and an appropriate educational programme that will help the child realise their potential.

Any intra-brain procedure is frightening for the family. Parents'/guardians' knowledge on the human anatomy and physiology may not be very good. So it is important that, before discharge, the anatomy and physiology of the nervous system is explained in a manner that the family can understand. They must know how to look after a child with a shunt. If the pump is not automatic, they must know how and when to open the valve so that they do not cause a mechanical obstruction because of lack of knowledge. This skill must be mastered before the child is discharged. They need to know the signs of obstruction, malfunctioning and infection of the shunt. These include poor feeding, headache, nausea and vomiting, increased temperature, abdominal distension, decreasing level of consciousness and seizures. They must understand that the shunt has to be changed as the child grows. Contact sport must be avoided, as the child may fall or be bumped. This will damage the shunt or dislodge the insertion point. It is recommended that the child wears a helmet to avoid injury and damage to the shunt.

The family and the child need to be enrolled with a support group for hydrocephalus sufferers where they will meet other people living with the condition and be able to share experiences, coping mechanisms and skills.

Conclusion

Hydrocephalus, whether congenital or acquired, is a very difficult condition to manage. The prognosis depends on the degree of brain damage before the shunt. Many have a high incidence of neurologically disabling challenges.

Suggested activities for learners

Activity 11.1
- Explain the pathophysiology of hydrocephalus including the clinical manifestation
- Explain the care of a child with a ventriculoperitoneal shunt at home.

References

Harrison, V. 2012. *The newborn baby*. 6th edition. Cape Town: Juta.

Hockenberry, MJ, & Wilson, D. 2015. *Wong's nursing care of infants and children*. 10th edition. Elsevier.

Mogotlane, S, Mokoena, J, Chauke, M, Matlakala, M, Young, A, & Randa, B. 2018. *Juta's complete textbook of medical surgical nursing*. 2nd edition. Cape Town: Juta.

Mott, SR, James, SR, & Sperhac, AM. 1990. *Nursing care of children and families*. 2nd edition. New York: Addison-Wesley Nursing.

Addendum A

Guidelines on basic care provisions in surgical wards and paediatric units

Checklist for PO5 Surgical Ward

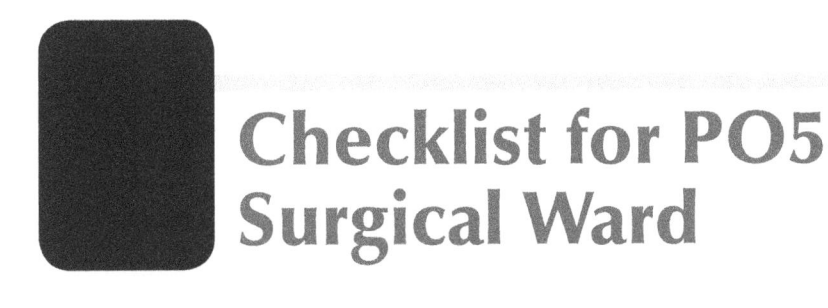

CHECKLIST DOMAIN 1 – PATIENT RIGHTS
1.2 Access to information for patients
Parents/guardians are provided with information to enable them to make informed decisions regarding their child's care.

Number of checklist	Criterion	Checklist reference	Measure
1.2.1.2.2	The correct procedure is followed to ensure that parents/patients give informed consent.	Consent forms in files	Forms used for informed consent are completed correctly by the health professionals
Number of questions	**Planned number of responses**	**Unit where assessed**	**Type of assessment**
9	5	P07/P05/P10/PC01/PX10	PRA

Instructions: Informed consent needs to apply to a variety of procedures, including HIV tests; PCR; clinical procedures in the health establishment. Check 3 files, from any of the units: HIV/AIDS clinic, surgical and one other, preferably those where the patient is present so the assessor can check on point 2 and 3. Mark yes or no

No.	Question/aspect	Patient 1 YES	Patient 1 NO	Patient 2 YES	Patient 2 NO	Patient 3 YES	Patient 3 NO	Comments
1	Check that the patient was legally entitled to give informed consent							
2	The doctor/nurse doing the procedure has appropriately completed the informed consent form							
3	The exact nature of the operation/procedure/treatment is written on the consent form							
4	The patient's full names are written on the consent form							
5	The consent form is signed by the patient or parent/guardian as appropriate for children							
6	The consent form is signed by the healthcare provider performing the procedure							
7	The consent form is signed by two witnesses							
8	The consent form is dated							
9	The above information is legible							
Actual score (sum of positive responses)								
Maximum possible score (sum of all questions minus the not applicable responses)								

CHECKLIST DOMAIN 1 – PATIENT RIGHTS
1.2 Access to information for patients
Patients are provided with information to enable them to make informed decisions regarding their care

Number of checklist	Criterion	Checklist reference	Measure
1.2.1.3.1	Patients are provided with a discharge report at the time of discharge as required by the National Health Act 61 of 2003	Discharge summary	3 files of discharged patients reflect a discharge summary report, which is completed comprehensively
Number of questions	**Planned number of responses**	**Unit where assessed**	**Type of assessment**
9	3	P04/P05/P06/PX03/PX04/PX05/PX06	PRA

Instructions: Check the files of 3 patients who have been discharged if they contain the details listed below. If the information is written in the discharge summary, allocate a 1, if not allocate a 0.

No.	Question/aspect	File 1 Yes	File 1 No	File 2 Yes	File 2 No	File 3 Yes	File 3 No	Comment
1	Date of admission							
2	Date of discharge							
3	Reason for admission/consultation							
4	Treating unit							
5	Diagnosis on discharge							
6	Medication and treatment given (including procedures and a description of laboratory tests, if appropriate)							
7	Follow-up instruction at the clinic/hospital							
8	Details of referrals and/or follow-up appointments							
9	Signature of healthcare provider							
Actual score (sum of positive responses)								
Maximum possible score (sum of all questions minus the not applicable responses)								

CHECKLIST DOMAIN 2 – PATIENT SAFETY
2.4 Clinical risk
Specific safety protocols are in place for high-risk groups of patients.

Number of checklist	Criterion	Checklist reference	Measure
2.4.3.2.1	Appropriate safety measures are implemented in the operating theatre before and during surgery	Perioperative document check	Patient perioperative document demonstrates that safety checks have been conducted during and after surgery as per WHO guidelines
Number of questions	**Planned number of responses**	**Unit where assessed**	**Type of assessment**
12	54	P05/P10/PX05/PX10	PRA

Instructions: Analyse the perioperative documents of 3 patients having operations and check that each aspect listed below is adhered to. If the factor has been assessed, mark Y for yes, if not, mark N for no.

No.	Question/aspect	1	2	3	Comments
	Before induction of anaesthesia:				
1	Patient's identity confirmed				
2	Patient procedure and site confirmed				
3	Patient consent confirmed				
4	Site marked				
	Precautions taken to maintain skin integrity				
	Baseline vital signs – pre anaesthesia				
5	Anaesthesia safety check completed				
6	Pulse oximeter on patient and functioning				
7	Was the patient checked for allergies?				
8	Does the patient have a difficult airway?				
9	Is there a record made of estimated blood loss?				
	Before skin incision:				
1	Confirm all team members have introduced themselves and their roles				
2	Surgeon, anaesthetist and nurse verbally confirm patient, site and procedure				
3	Any anticipated critical events noted and documented				
4	Has antibiotic prophylaxis been given?				
	Before patient leaves the operating room:				
1	Nurse to verbally confirm the name of the procedure				

2	Nurse to verbally confirm that instrument, sponge and needle counts are correct			
3	Was the specimen labeled?			
4	Are any equipment problems to be addressed?			
5	Surgeon, anaesthetist and nurse confirm key concerns for recovery and management of the patient			
Actual score (sum of positive responses)				
Maximum possible score (sum of all questions minus the not applicable responses)				

CHECKLIST DOMAIN 2 – PATIENT SAFETY
2.4 Clinical risk
Specific safety protocols are in place for high-risk groups of patients.

Number of checklist	Criterion	Checklist reference	Measure
2.4.3.3.4 & 2.4.3.3.5	The safety of patients who require resuscitation is assured	Emergency trolleys	Emergency trolleys are standardised, appropriately stocked and regularly checked
Number of questions	**Planned number of responses**	**Unit where assessed**	**Type of assessment**
26	26	P07/P10/P01/P02/P09 MC14/MC14A/PX01/ PX09/PX07	OBS

Instructions: Check the contents of the emergency trolley against the list below. Ask if the equipment is functional and assign Y for yes and N for No. Only for the highlighted equipment check if an operator's manual is available.
Only for the highlighted equipment check if the consumables used in the equipment's operations is available.

No.	Question/aspect	Functional Yes	Not functional No	Comments
	EXTREME MEASURES			
1	AED machine/ECG monitor/defibrillator, pads, paddles and electrodes			
2	Laryngoscope with blades (adults + paeds)			
3	Tracheal tubes adult as appropriate			
4	Tracheal tubes paediatric as appropriate			
5	Manual resuscitator device/ambubag (adult)			
6	Manual resuscitator device/ambubag (paeds)			
7	Oxygen masks and/or nasal cannula (adults + paeds)			
8	Emergency medications that have not expired, according to local protocol			
9	AED and emergency trolley are checked on a daily basis			
Actual score (sum of positive responses)				
Maximum possible score (sum of all questions minus the not applicable responses)				

No.	Question/aspect	Functional Yes	Not functional No	Comments
	EXTREME MEASURES			
1	Universal precautions equipment (gloves, eye protection, face mask)			
2	Blood pressure cuffs			
3	Glucometer			
4	Thermometer			
5	Pulse oximeter			
6	Scissors			
7	Oropharyngeal airways/nasopharyngeal airways			
8	Laryngeal mask airways			
9	Xylocaine spray			
10	KY jelly/Remicaine gel			
11	ET tube – plaster/tie to secure (adult + paed)			
12	Magill forceps (adults + paed)			
13	Nasogastric tubes (adults + paed)			
14	Oxygen supply ready for use (portable or fixed unit)			
15	Suction catheters (6F to 14F)			
16	Suction devices (portable or fixed power)			
Actual score (sum of positive responses)				
Maximum possible score (sum of all questions minus the not applicable responses)				

CHECKLIST DOMAIN 2 – PATIENT SAFETY
2.4 Clinical risk
Specific safety protocols are in place for high-risk groups of patients.

Number of checklist	Criterion	Checklist reference	Measure
2.4.3.5.1	Blood and blood products are administered so as to protect patients from harm	Guidelines for the safe administration of blood and blood products	Patient files demonstrate that the protocol on administration of blood has been adhered to
Number of questions	**Planned number of responses**	**Unit where assessed**	**Type of assessment**
16	16	PO1/PO5/PX01/PX05	PRA

Instructions: Check the files of 3 patients for compliance with the protocol on administration of blood and blood products and check that each of the aspects listed below is included in the record. If the factor has been assessed, mark Y for yes, if not, mark N for no.

No.	Question/aspect	Patient 1	Patient 2	Patient 3	Comments
1	The clinical need for blood is documented				
2	Informed consent from patient is documented				
3	Selection of blood product required is documented				

4	Checks were conducted prior to administration of blood, which included: Checking the identity of the patient		
5	Checking the product		
6	Checking the patient's documentation		
7	Patient's vitals were monitored prior, during administration and for 12 hours after		
8	Recording details of the transfusion		
Actual score (sum of positive responses)			
Maximum possible score (sum of all questions minus the not applicable responses)			

CHECKLIST DOMAIN 2 – PATIENT SAFETY
2.5 Adverse events
Adverse events are identified and promptly responded to, to reduce patient harm and suffering.

Number of checklist	Criterion	Checklist reference	Measure
2.5.1.2.1	The establishment actively encourages a culture of effective reporting of adverse events	Culture	2 staff members interviewed to confirm that the health establishment encourages the reporting of adverse events
Number of questions	Planned number of responses	Unit where assessed	Type of assessment
4	8	P04/P05/P06/P07/PX07/ PX04/PX05/PX06 MC14/MC14A	SI

Instructions: Interview 2 staff members and check if they are comfortable to report adverse events and what management's attitude is towards adverse events. Mark Y for yes or N for no.

No.	Question/aspect	Staff 1	Staff 2
1	Are you comfortable to report adverse events?		
2	Does management accept your adverse events report?		
3	Does management use the reports to improve patient care?		
4	Does management encourage you to report events?		
Actual score (sum of positive responses)			
Maximum possible score (sum of all questions minus the not applicable responses)			

CHECKLIST DOMAIN 2 – PATIENT SAFETY
2.6 Infection prevention and control
Universal precautions are applied to prevent healthcare-associated infections.

Number of checklist	Criterion	Checklist reference	Measure
2.6.3.2.1	Sharps are safely managed and disposed of	Universal precautions policy	A random selection of 3 clinical areas: show that sharps and needles are disposed of safely

Number of questions	Planned number of responses	Unit where assessed	Type of assessment
4	12	P10/P06/P09/P04/P05/PX10/PX06/PX04/PX05/PX07 MC14/MC14A/PC01	OBS

Instructions: Randomly select 3 clinical areas to observe whether sharps, needles and collection of sharps are correctly managed.
Do staff do the following (mark Y for yes or N for no)?

No.	Question/aspect	Area 1	Area 2	Area 3	Comments
1	Do the staff observe safe practices in the disposal of sharps and needles?				
2	Observe for the quality and availability of sharps containers				
3	Available containers have correctly fitting lids				
4	Staff recap needles before disposal and dispose of syringes with the attached needle in their entirety				
Actual score (sum of positive responses)					
Maximum possible score (sum of all questions minus the not applicable responses)					

CHECKLIST DOMAIN 3 – CLINICAL SUPPORT SERVICES
3.2 Diagnostic services
Accessible and effective laboratory services enhance patient diagnosis.

Number of checklist	Criterion	Checklist reference	Measure
3.2.1.1.3	Laboratory services are available and results are provided within agreed-upon turnaround times	Available times for test results	Laboratory results requested are available in 3 of the patients' files

Number of questions	Planned number of responses	Unit where assessed	Type of assessment

| 3 | 3 | C07/C09/C10/MC14/ MC14A/MX07/MX09 | DA |

Instructions: Randomly select 3 files/records and check whether most recently ordered laboratory test results are available in the patient's file. Tick the Yes column if they are and the No column if they are not.

	Yes	No	Comments
Patient file 1			
Patient file 2			
Patient file 3			
Actual score (sum of positive responses)			
Maximum possible score (sum of all questions minus the not applicable responses)			

CHECKLIST DOMAIN 6

6.7 Medical records

Individual patient information is accurately and completely recorded according to clinical, legal and ethical requirements.

Number of checklist	Criterion	Checklist reference	Measure
6.7.1.1.1	Patient records are complete and contain all legal and statutory requirements	Medical records	2 patient files comply with legal and statutory requirements for record-keeping
Number of questions	**Planned number of responses**	**Unit where assessed**	**Type of assessment**
23	46	P03/P04/P05/P06/P09/ MC14/MC14A/PX03/PX04/ PX05/PX06/PX09	PRA

Instruction: Request the records of 2 patients to check for compliance with record-keeping. Tick in the Yes column for yes and
No column for no.

No.	Question/aspect	Yes	No	Comments
1	Patient's name and address are recorded			
2	Patient's date of birth and age recorded			
3	Hospital/clinic number recorded			
4	Contact details of next of kin recorded			
5	Home language recorded			
6	Results of investigations in record			
7	Doctor/nurse has recorded his qualifications against entries			
8	Doctor/nurse has recorded date and time against entries			
9	Doctor/nurse has signed entries			
10	Name/signature is legible in records			
11	Discharge summary in file			

12	ICD 10 coding is completed	
13	Procedure coding is completed	
14	Daily day-time progress notes made	
15	Daily night-time progress notes made	
16	Balfec chart for fluid monitoring completed and in file	
17	Nursing care plan complete and in file	
18	Medicine administration chart in file. Medications administered signed, dated and time recorded, dosage reflected, dosage frequency	
19	Only authorised abbreviations used	
20	All records are legible	
21	All entries are in black ink	
22	All entries are dated and time recorded	
23	Each entry made by a health professional is signed	
Actual score (sum of positive responses)		
Maximum possible score (sum of all questions minus the not applicable responses)		

CHECKLIST DOMAIN 7 – FACILITIES AND INFRASTRUTURE

7.4 Hygiene and cleanliness

The buildings and grounds are kept clean and hygienic to maximise safety and comfort.

Number of checklist	Criterion	Checklist reference	Measure
7.4.1.2.1	Appropriate cleaning materials and equipment are available and properly used and stored	Cleanliness	Cleaning materials cloths/dusters/scourers and chemicals and equipment are available and stored in an appropriate safe lockable area, with clear labels for equipment used internally and externally

Number of questions	Planned number of responses	Unit where assessed	Type of assessment
23	23	SO2/PCO8/PO7-2/PO9/ PO10-1/PO11/P11/P12/ P13/SO2/PO4-2/PO5-2/ P10-2/PO1/PO2/PO3/PO5	OBS

Instructions: Assess the area for cleaning materials and storage facility. Tick the Yes column if the elements are present and the No column if they are not. Mark N/A if item is not part of routine supplies in facility.

	SPECIFY AREA										
No.	Question/aspect	Yes	No	Yes	No	Yes	No	Yes	No	Yes	No	Comments
1	Does the toilet and/or bathroom appear clean?										

2	**Hand hygiene for cleaning staff**	
2.1	Plain liquid soap or non-antimicrobial soap	
2.2	Alcohol-based hand rub with emollient	
2.3	Antimicrobial soap	
2.4	Disposable sponges	
2.5	Paper towels	
3	**Personal protective equipment for cleaning staff**	
3.1	Gloves (non-sterile and sterile)	
3.2	Long-sleeve gowns/disposable aprons	
3.3	Surgical masks (face covers)	
3.4	Particulate masks (N-95 respirator)	
3.5	Goggles	
3.6	Face shields (visors)	
4	**Cleaning of the environment and general cleaning**	
4.1	Water and detergent-based solutions	
4.2	Janitor trolley	
4.3	Colour-coded buckets and cloths	
4.4	Spray bottle (containing dishwashing detergent/disinfectant solution)	
4.5	Window cleaning squeegee	

4.6	Mop sweeper or soft-platform broom	
4.7	Protective polymer	
4.8	Wet vacuum pick up	
5	**Waste management supplies on the cleaning trolley or in the supplies/ storage area**	
5.1	Red bags	
5.2	Yellow bags	
5.3	Black bags	
5.4	Sealed impervious containers for waste disposal	
5.5	Are cleaning materials stored in an appropriate safe lockable area?	
Actual score (sum of positive responses)		
Maximum possible score (sum of all questions minus the not applicable responses)		

Checklist for PO6 Paediatric Ward

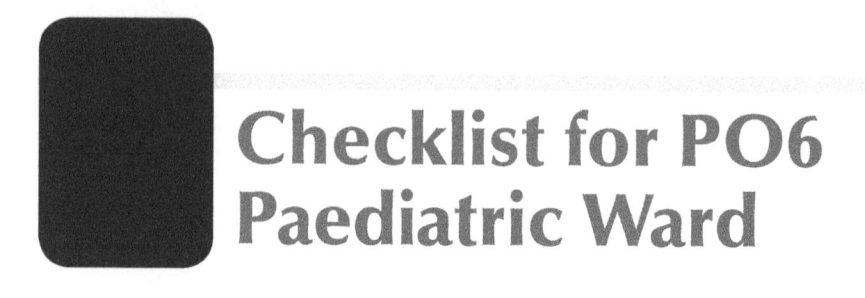

CHECKLIST DOMAIN 1 – PATIENT RIGHTS

1.2 Access to information for patients

Patients are provided with information to enable them to make informed decisions regarding their care.

Number of checklist	Criterion	Checklist reference	Measure
1.2.1.3.1	Patients are provided with a discharge report at the time of discharge as required by the National Health Act 61 of 2003	Discharge summary	3 files of discharged patients reflect a discharge summary report, which is completed comprehensively

Number of questions	Planned number of responses	Unit where assessed	Type of assessment
9	3	PO4/PO5/PO6/PX03/PX04/PX05/PX06	PRA

Instructions: Check the files of 3 patients who have been discharged if they contain the details listed below. If the information is written in the discharge summary, allocate a 1, if not allocate a 0.

No.	Question/aspect	File 1 Yes	File 1 No	File 2 Yes	File 2 No	File 3 Yes	File 3 No	Comment
1	Date of admission							
2	Date of discharge							
3	Reason for admission/consultation							
4	Treating unit							
5	Diagnosis on discharge							
6	Medication and treatment given (including procedures and a description of laboratory tests, if appropriate)							
7	Follow-up instruction at the clinic/hospital							
8	Details of referrals and/or follow-up appointments							
9	Signature of healthcare provider							
	Actual score (sum of positive responses)							
	Maximum possible score (sum of all questions minus the not applicable responses)							

CHECKLIST DOMAIN 2 – PATIENT SAFETY

2.1 Patient care

The basic care and treatment of patients contributes to positive health outcomes.

Number of checklist	Criterion	Checklist reference	Measure
2.1.1.1.1	Procedures are in place to deliver basic care that contributes to positive health outcomes	Clinical assessment and diagnosis	The files of 3 patients who have been discharged in the past 24 hours show that a comprehensive clinical assessment and diagnosis has been done
Number of questions	**Planned number of responses**	**Unit where assessed**	**Type of assessment**
9	27	P07/PC01	PRA

Instructions: Take 3 files of patients who have been recently discharged from the ward and check that the following aspects were done. It is assumed that if the doctor/PHC nurse has not written that they did the examination, etc., it was not done. For PHC clinics, check 3 random files. Allocate Y for yes and N for no.

No.	Question/aspect	Patient 1 Yes	Patient 1 No	Patient 2 Yes	Patient 2 No	Patient 3 Yes	Patient 3 No
1	The past medical history was asked and noted						
2	The notes indicate that a physical examination of the patient was done, including vitals taken						
3	The notes state a provisional diagnosis after initial assessment						
4	There is a plan of treatment noted by the doctor/PHC nurse						
5	There is a plan of treatment noted by the nurse/PHC nurse						
6	There is evidence that the patient was informed about the treatment and given health education						
7	There is evidence that the doctor/PHC nurse examined the patient at least on the day of or before discharge						
8	The notes state that a discharge diagnosis was made						
9	The notes state that a plan for treatment and follow-up care was made						
Actual score (sum of positive responses)							
Maximum possible score (sum of all questions minus the not applicable responses)							

CHECKLIST DOMAIN 2 – PATIENT SAFETY
2.4 Clinical risk
Specific safety protocols are in place for high-risk groups of patients

Number of checklist	Criterion	Checklist reference	Measure
2.4.3.3.4 & 2.4.3.3.5	The safety of patients who require resuscitation is assured	Emergency trolleys	Emergency trolleys are standardised, appropriately stocked and regularly checked
Number of questions	**Planned number of responses**	**Unit where assessed**	**Type of assessment**
26	26	P07/P10/P01/P02/P09 MC14/MC14A/ PX01/PX09/PX07	OBS

Instructions: Check the contents of the emergency trolley against the list below. Ask if the equipment is functional and assign Y for yes and N for no. Only for the highlighted equipment check if an operator's manual is available.
Only for the highlighted equipment check if the consumables used in the equipment's operations is available.

No.	Question/aspect	Functional Yes	Not functional No	Comments
	EXTREME MEASURES			
1	AED machine/ECG monitor/defibrillator, pads, paddles and electrodes			
2	Laryngoscope with blades (adults + paeds)			
3	Tracheal tubes adult as appropriate			
4	Tracheal tubes Paediatric as appropriate			
5	Manual resuscitator device/ambubag (adult)			
6	Manual resuscitator device/ambubag (paeds)			
7	Oxygen masks and/or nasal cannula (adults + paeds)			
8	Emergency medications that have not expired, according to local protocol			
9	AED and emergency trolley are checked on a daily basis			

Actual score (sum of positive responses) HIGH RISK MEASURES

Maximum possible score (sum of all questions minus the not applicable responses)

No.	Question/aspect	Functional Yes	Not functional No	Comments
	EXTREME MEASURES			
1	Universal precautions equipment (gloves, eye protection, face mask)			
2	Blood pressure cuffs			
3	Glucometer			
4	Thermometer			
5	Pulse oximeter			
6	Scissors			

7	Oropharyngeal airways/nasopharyngeal airways	
8	Laryngeal mask airways	
9	Xylocaine spray	
10	KY jelly/Remicaine gel	
11	ET tube – plaster/tie to secure (adult + paed)	
12	Magill forceps (adults + paed)	
13	Nasogastric tubes (adults + paed)	
14	Oxygen supply ready for use (portable or fixed unit)	
15	Suction catheters (6F to 14F)	
16	Suction devices (portable or fixed power)	
Actual score (sum of positive responses)		
Maximum possible score (sum of all questions minus the not applicable responses)		

CHECKLIST DOMAIN 2 – PATIENT SAFETY
2.4 Clinical risk
Specific safety protocols are in place for high-risk groups of patients.

Number of checklist	Criterion	Checklist reference	Measure
2.4.3.4.2	The safety of patients receiving medication is assured	Safe administration of medicine	Observation of 3 patients receiving medication confirms that patients' safety is assured
Number of checklist	**Planned number of responses**	**Unit where assessed**	**Type of assessment**
7	27	P07/P06/PX06/PX07/PC01	OBS

Instructions: Observe a nurse in the ward or clinic giving out medicines to patients. Check that they adhere to all the aspects listed below for each patient. If the factor has been assessed, mark Y for yes and N for no.
The assessor may wish to ask the nurse to explain what they are doing to understand whether or not they are adhering to the requirements.

No.	Question/aspect	1	2	3	Comments
	The nurse checks that:				
1	The right medicine is given				
2	The container label is clear and visible				
3	The medicine is given at the right time				
4	The right dose of medicine is given, including the measurement of the dose				
5	The right route is used				
6	The right patient received the medicine				
7	Has patient been observed to take medication, including swallowing?				
8	Does the nurse explain to the patient/guardian how to administer the medicine at home?				

9	Does the nurse explain to the patient/guardian what the side effects are and what to do in case of side effects?		
Actual score (sum of positive responses)			
Maximum possible score (sum of all questions minus the not applicable responses)			

CHECKLIST DOMAIN 2 – PATIENT SAFETY
2.5 Adverse events

Adverse events are identified and promptly responded to, to reduce patient harm and suffering.

Number of checklist	Criterion	Checklist reference	Measure
2.5.1.2.1	The establishment actively encourages a culture of effective reporting of adverse events	Culture	2 staff members interviewed to confirm that the health establishment encourages the reporting of adverse events

Number of questions	Planned number of responses	Unit where assessed	Type of assessment
4	8	P04/P05/P06/P07/PX07/PX04/PX05/PX06/MC14/MC14A	SI

Instructions: Interview 2 staff members and check if they are comfortable to report adverse events and what management's attitude is towards adverse events. Mark Y for yes or N for no.

No.	Question/aspect	Staff 1	Staff 2
1	Are you comfortable to report adverse events?		
2	Does management accept your adverse events report?		
3	Does management use the reports to improve patient care?		
4	Does management encourage you to report events?		
Actual score (sum of positive responses)			
Maximum possible score (sum of all questions minus the not applicable responses)			

CHECKLIST DOMAIN 2 – PATIENT SAFETY
2.6 Infection prevention and control

Universal precautions are applied to prevent healthcare-associated infections.

Number of checklist	Criterion	Checklist reference	Measure
2.6.3.2.1	Sharps are safely managed and disposed of	Universal precautions policy	A random selection of 3 clinical areas: show that sharps and needles are disposed of safely

Checklist for PO6 Paediatric Ward

Number of checklist	Planned number of responses	Unit where assessed	Type of assessment
4	12	P10/P06/P09/P04/P05 PX10/PX06/PX04/PX05/PX07 MC14/MC14A/PC01	OBS

Instructions: Randomly select 3 clinical areas to observe whether sharps, needles and collection of sharps are correctly managed.
Do staff do the following (mark Y for yes or N for no)?

No.	Question/aspect	Area 1	Area 2	Area 3	Comments
1	Do the staff observe safe practices in the disposal of sharps and needles?				
2	Observe for the quality and availability of sharps containers				
3	Available containers have correctly fitting lids				
4	Staff recap needles before disposal and dispose of syringes with the attached needle in their entirety				
Actual score (sum of positive responses)					
Maximum possible score (sum of all questions minus the not applicable responses)					

CHECKLIST DOMAIN 3 – CLINICAL SUPPORT SERVICES
3.2 Diagnostic services

Accessible and effective laboratory services enhance patient diagnosis.

Number of checklist	Criterion	Checklist reference	Measure
3.2.1.1.3	Laboratory services are available and results are provided within agreed-upon turnaround times	Available times for test results	Laboratory results requested are available in 3 of the patients' files

Number of questions	Planned number of responses	Unit where assessed	Type of assessment
3	3	C07/C09/C10/MC14/ MC14A/MX07/MX09	DA

Instructions: Randomly select 3 files/records and check whether most recently ordered laboratory test results are available in the patient's file. Tick the Yes column if they are and the No column if they are not.

		Yes	No	Comments
	Patient file 1			
	Patient file 2			
	Patient file 3			
Actual score (sum of positive responses)				
Maximum possible score (sum of all questions minus the not applicable responses)				

CHECKLIST DOMAIN 4

4.2 Health promotion and disease prevention

The importance of health promotion and disease prevention as part of patient care is actively promoted and practised.

Number of checklist	Criterion	Checklist reference	Measure
4.2.1.1.1	The health establishment delivers and monitors primary prevention programmes for at-risk patients to impact on the determinants of health	Primary Prevention Programmes	3 randomly selected patient files 1. Antenatal card (ANC) 2. Immunisation 3. IMCI 4. TB/HIV 5. Non-communicable disease Indicates that primary prevention programmes were delivered.

Number of questions	Planned number of responses	Unit where assessed	Type of assessment
11	15	P06/P03/PC01	PRA

Instructions: Randomly select 3 patient files as listed and respond to following questions. Allocate a Y for yes and a N for a no.

No.	Question/aspect	Yes	No	Comments
1. ANC	Was HIV Counselling and Testing (HCT) offered to the patient?			
	Was the Blood Pressure (BP) of the patient monitored every visit?			
2. Immunisation	Is the immunisation up-to-date according to the child's age?			
	Was the child weighed with every visit?			
3. IMCI	Has the child received Mebendasole for de-worming?			
	Was Vitamin A given to the child as per schedule?			
4. TB/HIV	Was TB patient counselled and tested for HIV?			
	Was the TB-positive patient advised and placed on Direct Observation of Treatment (DOTS)?			
	Has the CD4 count of the HIV-positive patient been done?			
5. Non-communicable disease	Is patient part of a support group?			
	Was health education given to the patient on preventing secondary illnesses?			
Actual score (sum of positive responses)				
Maximum possible score (sum of all questions minus the not applicable responses)				

CHECKLIST DOMAIN 6
6.7 Medical records

Individual patient information is accurately and completely recorded according to clinical, legal and ethical requirements.

Number of checklist	Criterion	Checklist reference	Measure
6.7.1.1.1	Patient records are complete and contain all legal and statutory requirements	Medical records	2 patient files comply with legal and statutory requirements for record-keeping

Number of checklist	Planned number of responses	Unit where assessed	Type of assessment
23	46	P03/P04/P05/P06/P09/MC14/MC14A/PX03/PX04/PX05/PX06/PX09	PRA

Instruction: Request the records of 2 patients for compliance with record-keeping. Tick the Yes column for yes and the No column for no.

No.	Question/aspect	Yes	No	Comments
1	Patient's name and address are recorded			
2	Patient's date of birth and age recorded			
3	Hospital/clinic number recorded			
4	Contact details of next of kin recorded			
5	Home language recorded			
6	Results of investigations in record			
7	Doctor/nurse has recorded his qualifications against entries			
8	Doctor/nurse has recorded date and time against entries			
9	Doctor/nurse has signed entries			
10	Name/signature is legible in records			
11	Discharge summary in file			
12	ICD 10 coding is completed			
13	Procedure coding is completed			
14	Daily day-time progress notes made			
15	Daily night-time progress notes made			
16	Balfec chart for fluid monitoring completed and in file			
17	Nursing care plan complete and in file			
18	Medicine administration chart in file. Medications administered signed, dated and time recorded, dosage reflected, dosage frequency			
19	Only authorised abbreviations used			
20	All records are legible			

21	All entries are in black ink		
22	All entries are dated and time recorded		
23	Each entry made by a health professional is signed		
Actual score (sum of positive responses)			
Maximum possible score (sum of all questions minus the not applicable responses)			

CHECKLIST DOMAIN 7 – FACILITIES AND INFRASTRUTURE
7.4 Hygiene and cleanliness

The buildings and grounds are kept clean and hygienic to maximise safety and comfort.

Number of checklist	Criterion	Checklist reference	Measure
7.4.1.2.1	Appropriate cleaning materials and equipment are available and properly used and stored	Cleanliness	Cleaning materials cloths/dusters/scourers and chemicals and equipment are available and stored in an appropriate safe lockable area, with clear labels for equipment used internally and externally

Number of questions	Planned number of responses	Unit where assessed	Type of assessment
23	23	SO2/PCO8/PO7-2/ PO9/PO10-1/PO11/ P11/P12/P13/SO2/ PO4-2/PO5-2/P10-2/ PO1/PO2/PO3/PO5	OBS

Instructions: Assess the area for cleaning materials and storage facility. Tick the Yes column if the elements are present and the No column if they are not. Mark N/A if item is not part of routine supplies in facility.

No	SPECIFY AREA Question/aspect	Yes	No	Yes	No	Yes	No	Yes	No	Yes	No	Comments
1	Does the toilet and/or bathroom appear clean?											
2	Hand hygiene for cleaning staff											
2.1	Plain liquid soap or non-antimicrobial soap											
2.2	Alcohol-based hand rub with emollient											
2.3	Antimicrobial soap											
2.4	Disposable sponges											
2.5	Paper towels											
3	Personal protective equipment for cleaning staff											
3.1	Gloves (non-sterile and sterile)											
3.2	Long-sleeve gowns/disposable aprons											

3.3	Surgical masks (face covers)	
3.4	Particulate masks (N-95 respirator)	
3.5	Goggles	
3.6	Face shields (visors)	
4	**Cleaning of the environment and general cleaning**	
4.1	Water and detergent-based solutions	
4.2	Janitor trolley	
4.3	Colour-coded buckets and cloths	
4.4	Spray bottle (containing dish washing detergent/disinfectant solution)	
4.5	Window cleaning squeegee	
4.6	Mop sweeper or soft-platform broom	
4.7	Protective polymer	
4.8	Wet vacuum pick up	
5	**Waste management supplies on the cleaning trolley or in the supplies/storage area**	
5.1	Red bags	
5.2	Yellow bags	
5.3	Black bags	
5.4	Sealed impervious containers for waste disposal	
5.5	Are cleaning materials stored in an appropriate safe lockable area?	
Actual score (sum of positive responses)		
Maximum possible score (sum of all questions minus the not applicable responses)		

Index

Page numbers in *italics* indicate where you will find information in figures or tables.

A

ablative surgery 29
abnormality, *see* acquired abnormality; congenital abnormality
absence of body parts, *see* congenital absence of body parts
access to information
 paediatric ward 162
 surgical ward 151–152
acquired abnormality 71
acquired defects 28
acute appendicitis, *see* appendicitis
adaptation 3
adenoidectomy 121
adenoids 122
adhesions
 definition 115
 wound infection 62
adverse events
 paediatric ward 166
 surgical ward 156
aganglionic megacolon 102
age
 cleft lip operation 73
 developmental milestones *8–10*
 preoperative risk factor 33
air conditioning 43
airway obstruction 59
airway patency 78
amputation 129, 137–138
anaesthesia
 checklist 31
 definition 41
anaesthetic nurse
 definition 41
 role of 46

anaesthetist 41
analgesic 55
aganglionic megacolon, *see* congenital aganglionic megacolon
anorexia 115
anxiety
 appendicectomy *119–120*
 cleft lip and cleft palate repair *79*
 congenital diaphragmatic hernia repair *95*
 fractured limb *140–141*
 oesophageal atresia repair *90–91*
 postoperative period *66–67*
 preoperative period 33
 types 110
APGAR score 83
appendicitis 115–120
aspiration 55
assent 25
ataxia 143
atelectasis 55

B

behavioural changes 21
bilateral long-leg hip spica cast *136*
birth history 32
bleeding (tracheostomy) 126
 see also haemorrhage
body jacket *136*
bone healing
 in children 131
 stages of 133
bone injury 130
 see also injury
buckle fracture *132*
burns 49

C

callus 129
callus formation 133
cardiac dysrhythmias 59
casts 134–136
cellular proliferation 133
cephalo-caudal 3
cerebrospinal fluid circulation *145*
cerebrospinal fluid (CSF) 144
checklist paediatric ward, *see* paediatric ward checklist
checklist surgical ward, *see* surgical ward checklist
child care
    growth and development 7
    parental involvement 6, 82
    risks involved 13–14
child (definition) 3
childhood morbidity 3
child mortality 3
children
    accident prone 13
    bone healing in 131
    fractures in 131
    gastrointestinal tract conditions 82
    intussusception in *98*
children in hospital
    adapting to hospital 18–19
    communicating information to 19
    informing of illness and treatment 6
    needs during surgery 29–30
    nursing assessment and findings 17–18
    own care 19
    pain 19–21, *see also* pain
    parental involvement 6, 82
    participation in care 19
    separation 14, 15
    trauma in 130
Children's Act The, *see* South African Children's Act
chronic tonsillitis 122
circulating nurse
    definition 41
    role of 45–46
cleft lip
    clinical manifestations 73
    nursing assessment 73
    nutrition 74
    pathophysiology 72–73
    postoperative care 74–75
    preoperative care 74
    preoperative risk factors 73–74
cleft palate 75–76
clinical risk
    paediatric ward 164–166
    surgical ward 153–155
closed cast 134
closed fracture 131
closed reduction 133
cognitive/problem solving *8–11*
colocolonic intussusception 98
comminuted fracture 131
community 8
complete fracture 130, *132*
compound fracture 131
congenital abnormality 71
congenital absence of body parts 137
congenital aganglionic megacolon 102–103
congenital defects 28, 72
    of the face 72–80
    of oesophageal and trachea 83–91
congenital diaphragmatic hernia
    assessment findings 92
    care 92–93
    clinical manifestations 92
    pathophysiology 91
    preparation for surgery 92
consciousness 143
consent
    common-law requirement for 14
    informed 13, 25
    invalid 39
    legal requirements 35–36
    operation 34–35
consent form 45
consolidation 133
constructive surgery 29
contamination 115
contractures 129, 136
corrective surgery 29
cosmetic surgery 29

coughing 60, 126
CSF, see cerebrospinal fluid
curative surgery 29

D
delayed union 136
denial stage 16
despair stage 15
detachment stage 16
development
   definition 3, 7
   and growth 6
   milestones in 8–11
diagnostic services
   paediatric ward 167
   surgical ward 157
diagnostic surgery 29
diaphragm 91
diaphragmatic hernia, see congenital diaphragmatic hernia
diaphysis 129
diet
   appendicectomy 119
   bringing food into hospital 17
   cleft lip and cleft palate 78
   postoperative 62, 64, 65
   surgery of the intestines 108, 110
disfigurement 141
distended bladder 63
due date 3
dysphagia 121

E
ectomy 28
elective surgery 29
elimination 59, 62
embryonic gut 82, 83
emergency surgery 29
epiphysis 129
ethical issues 34–36
exercise 62
exploratory surgery 29

F
falls 39
family
   definition 13
   health education 147–148
   heredity 7
   history 31
   socioeconomic environment 8
fine motor development 8–11
fluid deficit 58
fluid imbalance 50
fluid intake 29–30
fluid overload 53
foetus 3
follow-up visits 63
Food Safety Act of 1990 17
foregut 82
foreign objects 51–52
fractures
   classification 130
   clinical manifestations 131
   complications 136
   definition 129
   described in lines 130
   management 132–133
   postoperative care 136
   preoperative care 133
   reduction of 133
   types 131, 132
full-term infant 3

G
gametes 3
gape 55
gastrointestinal tract surgery 82
general anaesthesia 47
general health 33
greenstick fracture 132
gross motor development 8–11
growth 3
   definition 7
   and development 6–7
   factors influencing 7–8
guarding 115

H
haematoma formation 133
haemorrhage
   definition 121

fractured limb *139*
late postoperative period 61
postoperative period 58, *64–65*
post-tonsillectomy 124
surgery of the intestines *107–108*
tonsillectomy *125*
see also bleeding
health
essential information on 62
family education on 147-148
mother and child 8
preoperative 33
hernias 104–106
hiccups 55
high-Fowler's position 92
hindgut 83
hip spica *136*
Hirschsprung's disease 102–103
HIV status disclosure 14
hoarseness 121
hospital
assisting child to adapt 18–19
bringing food into 17
hospitalisation
assessment and findings 17–18
child's participation 19
child's reaction 15
coping with 18
definition 13
parents' reaction 16
parents' role 18
sibling participation 18–19
siblings' reaction 16–17
H-type link 84, 87
hydration
appendicectomy *119*
cleft lip and cleft palate repair *78–79*
congenital diaphragmatic hernia repair 95
oesophageal atresia repair *89–90*
preoperative period 33
types *109–110*
tonsillectomy *125*
hydrocephalus
clinical manifestations 144
definition 143

discharge plan 147–148
family education 147–148
postoperative care 147
preoperative care 146
types 144–146
hydrocephalus with the setting-sun sign *145*
hygiene and cleanliness
paediatric ward 170–171
surgical ward 159–161
hyperpyrexia 121
hypertension 59
hyperthermia 52
see also hypothermia
hypertrophic pyloric stenosis
care 97–98
clinical manifestations 96
signs of 97
hypervolaemia *53*
hypotension 59
hypothermia
intraoperative period 52
oesophageal atresia repair 90
postoperative period 59
hypovolaemia *52–53*
hypoxaemia 55, 59

I
ileocaecal intussusception 98, *99*
ileoileal intussusception 98
immobility *139*
impaired skin integrity *78*
imperforate anus 103–104
inadequate nutrition, *see under* nutrition
incomplete fracture 130
infant 4
infant mortality rate 4
infection
congenital diaphragmatic hernia repair 94
fractures 136, *139–140*
late postoperative period 61
oesophageal atresia repair 89
postoperative complication 147
postoperative period 60, *64*
post-tonsillectomy 124

surgery of the intestines 108–109
tonsillectomy 125
infection prevention and control
   paediatric ward 166–167
   surgical ward 156–157
informed consent, *see* consent
inguinal hernia 106
injury
   bones 130
   hernias 105
   intraoperative period 49, *51*
   tracheostomy 126
internal fixation 136
International Association of Study of Pain (IASP) 19
intracranial pressure 143
intraoperative nursing
   anaesthesia 47
   anaesthetic nurse 46
   cardiovascular complications 50
   care team 43–44
   circulating nurse 45–46
   complications 49–50
   consent form 45
   pain 50
   positioning of patient 47
   reception in operating room 46
   recovery room care 48–49
   return to ward 49
   scrub nurse 45
   theatre environment 42–43
   theatre reception nurse 44–45
intraoperative period 41
intussusception
   assessment findings 99
   care 99–100
   in children *98*
   clinical manifestations 99
   postoperative care problems 100
   recurrence 100
   types 98

J
Jehovah's Witness consent 26–27

K
keloid formation 62

L
language development *8–11*
large-for-dates 4
late postoperative-period care 61–62
lateral position 47
legal issues 34–36
lithotomy position 47
live birth 4
local anaesthesia 47
lodger mother 4
long arm cast *135*
long leg cast *135*
low birth weight 4
lumen 115

M
major surgery 29
malunion 136
maturation 4
medical records
   paediatric ward 169–170
   surgical ward 158–159
medication
   before anaesthesia 26
   calculation of dosages 6, 14, 32, 97
   upon discharge 62
   pain control 49, 55
   postoperative recovery 26
medico-legal hazards
   consent for surgery 36
   preoperative preparations 39
metaphysis 129
midgut 83
milestones 4, 8–11
minor surgery 28
mobility 62

N
nasogastric tube 92, 103
nausea
   appendicitis 116
   definition 115
   recovery room 50

neonatal mortality rate 4
neonatal period 4
non-curative surgery 29
non-union 136
nursing care plan
   appendicectomy *118–120*
   cleft lip and cleft palate *76–79*
   congenital diaphragmatic hernia *93–95*
   fractured limb *138–141*
   intraoperative period *50–53*
   oesophageal atresia *88–91*
   postoperative period *63–67*
   surgery of the intestines *107–110*
   tonsillectomy *124–125*
   tracheo-oesophageal fistula *88–91*
nutrition
   appendicectomy *119*
   before surgery 29–30, 33
   cleft lip repair 74, *78*
   cleft palate repair *78*
   diaphragmatic hernia repair *95*
   fractured limb *140*
   hernias 105
   inadequate 58
   oesophageal atresia repair *89–90*
   surgery of the intestines *109–110*
   tonsillectomy *125*

O
oblique fracture 130
obstetrics 32
obstruction
   airway 59, 126
   blood and lymph vessels 98
   Eustachian tube 122
   hypertrophic pyloric stenosis 96
   inguinal hernia 106
   intestinal 100, 101
   lumen 116
   oesophageal atresia 83
   shunts 147
   surgical removal 146
   tracheostomy 126, *127*
   volvulus 100
oesophageal atresia
   classification 85–87
   clinical manifestations 83–84
   permutations *84*
   postoperative care 87–88
   preoperative care 84
   types 83
oesophageal atresia with a fistula *86*
oesophageal atresia without fistula *85*
omphalocele hernia 104–105
one and one-half hip spica cast *136*
open cast 134
open complicated fracture 131
open reduction 133
operating room
   reception of patient in 46
   surgery 42
operation 4
opisthotonus 143
orrhaphy 28
oscopy 28
ossification 129, 133
osteoblasts 129
ostomy 28
otalgia 121
otomy 28

P
paediatrics 4, 6
paediatric ward checklist
   clinical support services 167
   facilities and infrastructure 170–171
   health promotion and disease prevention 168
   medical records 169–170
   patient rights 162
   patient safety 163–167
pain
   appendicectomy *118*
   assessment 20–21
   behavioural changes 21
   in children 19–21
   cleft lip and cleft palate repair *77–78*
   congenital diaphragmatic hernia repair *93*
   fractures 136, *138*
   intraoperative period *50–51*

postoperative period 58, *63*
psychological changes 21
questioning about 21
responses when in 21
surgery of the intestines *107*
tonsillectomy *124*
pain rating scales 20
palliative surgery 29
paralytic ileus 65–66, 100, *109*
parental involvement 6, 82
patient identification 39
patient management executives (PMEs) 44
patient teaching 124
perinatal mortality rate 4
perinatal period 5
perioperative documents 31
perioperative nursing care 25
periosteum 129
peritonitis *118–119*
peritonsillar abscess 124
permutations of oesophageal and tracheo-oesophageal defects *84*
phantom limb 129
phantom limb phenomenon 137
phantom pain 137
pharyngitis 121
pincer grip 5
plastic deformation *132*
plasty 28
pneumothorax 126
poly-hydramnios 5
postoperative care 25
postoperative medication 26
postoperative nursing
  care in ward 57–59
  subsequent care 59–60
  discharge preparations 62
  haemorrhage *64–65*
  hypothermia 59
  infection *64*
  pain 58
  preparation of environment 57
  problems 58–59, 62
postoperative period 55
post-term infant 5

post-tonsillectomy 124
premature infant 5
premedication 26, 37
premedication errors 39
preoperative nursing
  anxiety 33
  child's needs 29–30
  child visits 27
  definition 26
  hospitalisation 32–34
  indications for surgery 28
  legal and ethical issues 34–36
  nursing assessment 30–32
  risk factors 33–34
  surgical procedures 28
  theatre personnel visits 34
preoperative risk factors 33–34
pressure points 47
preterm infant, *see* premature infant
procedure
  extent of 34
  suffixes for surgical 28
projectile vomiting 96, 97
  see also vomiting
prone position 47
prophylactic surgery 29
prostatic pneumonia 60
prosthesis 129, 137
protest stage 15
proximo-distal 5
psychological care and comfort 30
psychological changes 21
psychological support 60
pulse oximeter 92
pyloric stenosis 96
pyloromyotomy 97
pylorus 96

Q
quinsy 121, 124

R
Ramstedt's procedure 97
reconstructive surgery 29
records, incorrect 39
recovery position *123*

recovery room care 48–49
reduced activity 60
reflex 143
regional anaesthesia 47
remodelling (bone) 133
respiratory distress 94
respiratory failure 88–89
rest and sleep 30

S
scrub nurse
    definition 41
    role of 45
self-care 62
separation 13
serious adverse event (SAE) 13
shivering 50
short arm cast 134
shoulder spica 135
shunts 147
shunt system 146
siblings 13
    managing of 17
    reaction to hospitalisation 16–17
simple fracture 131
singultus 55
site marking 30
skin incision 31
skin preparation 30, 39
skin status 131
small-for-dates 5
social emotions 8–11
South African Children's Act, The 38 of
    2005 3, 14
South African Patient's Rights Charter 26
speech development 8–11
spinal anaesthesia 47
spiral fracture 130
splint 129, 132
splinting devices 132
standard operating procedures (SOPs) 17
starving instructions 39
stillbirth 5
stillbirth rate 5
stump 130
supine position 47

surgery 5
    child's needs 29–30
    classification and types 28–29
    day of 37–38
    indications for 28
    nursing assessment 30–32
    as treatment option 27
surgical emphysema 126
surgical positions 47
surgical procedures 28
surgical ward checklist
    clinical support services 157
    facilities and infrastructure 159–161
    medical records 158–159
    patient rights 151–152
    patient safety 153–157
sutures 62
swelling 138

T
telephonic consent 35
temperature variation 50
tenderness 115
theatre environment 42–43
theatre reception area 41
theatre reception nurse 44–45
theatre recovery room 41
thumb spica 134
tonsillectomy 121, 122
tonsillitis
    assessment and findings 122
    patient teaching 124
    postoperative care 123–124
    preoperative care 122
    recovery position 123
tonsils 122
trachea 126
tracheal fistula 84, 87
tracheo-oesophageal fistula
    classification 85–87
    clinical manifestations 83–84
    permutations 84
    postoperative care 87–88
    preoperative care 84
    types 83
tracheooesophageal fistula 85

tracheooesophageal fistulae without atresia 86
tracheooesophageal fistula without atresia 87
tracheostomy 126–127
tracheostomy tube 127
transportation to operating theatre 37–38
transverse fracture 130
trimester 5

U
ulceration 115
umbilical hernia 105
unilateral hip spica cast 136

V
valuables 39
ventilatory complications 50
vital signs 39
volvulus 100–101
vomiting
  anaesthesia 47
  appendicitis 116

Hirschsprung's disease 102
hydrocephalus 146
hypertrophic pyloric stenosis 96, 97
intussusception 99
postoperative care 97
recovery room 50
volvulus 101

W
ward
  care upon arrival in 57–59
  returning patient to 49
  transportation from 37–38
warmth 30
weight loss 60
World Health Organization (WHO) guidelines 31
wound healing 61–62

Z
zygote 5

Lightning Source UK Ltd.
Milton Keynes UK
UKHW031829190721
387421UK00008B/1884

9 781485 115762